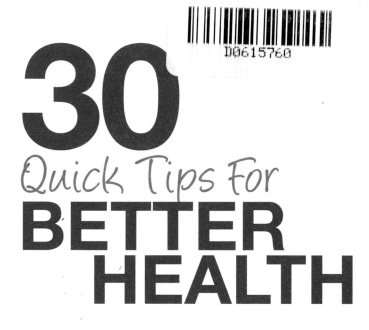

30
Quick Tips For
BETTER
HEALTH

DON VERHULST, MD

SILOAM

30 QUICK TIPS FOR BETTER HEALTH by Don VerHulst, MD
Published by Siloam
Charisma Media/Charisma House Book Group
600 Rinehart Road
Lake Mary, Florida 32746
www.charismahouse.com

Cover design by Lisa Rae Cox
Design Director: Bill Johnson

Visit the author's website at www.DrDonMD.com.

Library of Congress Cataloging-in-Publication Data:

VerHulst, Don.

  30 quick tips for better health : an easy-to-do guide to wellness / Don VerHulst.

      pages cm

  Summary: "People are bombarded with messages promoting unhealthy industrialized foods and lifestyles as well as messages telling them they need better nutrition and healthier lifestyles. 30 Quick Tips for Better Health provides the Bible's message on these important issues, broken down into thirty short, easy-to-read chapters that are easy to put into practice. With this quick guide to health, readers can use the book to build new wellness habits over a one-month period or leisurely read a lesson whenever they have time or need. Each of the thirty lessons is introduced by a Bible verse that serves as its basis"-- Provided by publisher.

  ISBN 978-1-62136-209-8 (pbk.) -- ISBN 978-1-62136-210-4 (e-book)

  1. Health. 2. Health--Religious aspects--Christianity. I. Title. II. Title: Thirty quick tips for better health.

  RA776.V41835 2013

  613--dc23

2012046130

First edition

13 14 15 16 17 — 9 8 7 6 5 4 3 2 1
Printed in the United States of America

Acknowledgments

I T IS WITH humble gratitude that I would like to acknowledge our pastor, Duane Vander Klok, for believing in my teaching gifts, and my colleague, Jim Bakker, for his support in embracing the Bible's message of health. I would also like to thank my friend and copy editor, E. M. Slootmaker, for her diligent, creative work as a wordsmith since this project first began.

Last but certainly not least, I praise the Lord for my loving family who continuously upholds me in my work—my dear mother, Jackquelyne VerHulst, for her support and cheerful willingness to care for our children when we are on the road with our ministry, and, most of all, my lovely wife, Susan Krews VerHulst. Without her hard work and attention to detail, this book would not have been possible.

—DR. DON VERHULST
PHILEMON 6

Contents

Introduction

TODAY IS A new day. What will you do with it? How about taking one step toward better health? In the following pages I will share some simple yet profound tips to help you live a healthier life—starting right now.

The Bible tells us in 3 John 2 that one of the things God most wants us to experience during our time here on earth is "good health" (NAS). Plenty of Scripture verses give us wisdom on good health. I will share that wisdom with you in this little book.

I also will provide you with practical action steps that will move you closer to optimum wellness. My prayer is that as you apply what you learn in this book, you will find yourself on the road to a healthier future.

You may already know some of the information you will read here. Perhaps you already include it as part of your lifestyle. I pray my words will then encourage you to stay the course. If this is all brand-new to you, I will show you some physical and spiritual changes you can make to look better, feel better, and have more energy.

Each of the thirty tips includes a specific Bible verse that gives health advice. After you read the verse and the health tip drawn from that passage of Scripture, pray for God to show you how to implement it in your life. Then record your thoughts and reactions in the space given for journaling and make a plan for how you can begin to make changes in your life—today.

As you read through this book, you'll quickly discover that the Bible is loaded with God's wisdom for improving your well-being. So I urge you to read these pages prayerfully, asking the

Holy Spirit to show you where change is needed. Then take at least one step to apply the truth of God's Word to your life. It will not only strengthen you spiritually, but it will also put you on the pathway to good health!

1   Read Your Owner's Manual

My son, attend to my words; consent and submit to my sayings. Let them not depart from your sight; keep them in the center of your heart. For they are life to those who find them, healing and health to all their flesh.

—PROVERBS 4:20–22

PROVERBS 4:20–22 GUARANTEES that God's words will be life to you—when you find them. Not only are they life, but they are also "health to all [your] flesh." The Hebrew word translated "health" in this passage can also mean "cure" or "remedy." God is saying His Word works as a medicine. But as with any medicine, you must take it as prescribed.

God has put a literal blueprint for your health within the pages of the Bible. If you want to be healthy, remember God's Word above all things!

The Bible is full of advice on how we should live here on earth. I think of it as a believer's owner's manual. When you buy a new car, bicycle, or toaster oven, do you read the owner's manual? If you're like most of us, you probably don't—until something goes wrong. But I'll bet you'd agree that you would be better prepared if you did read the manual as soon as you bought the new item, and that it's the best source for finding information on that product.

Your life is much more precious than any material thing you can buy. Take time to read your owner's manual every day. That way you will be prepared for any problems that come up in life—including health problems.

MAKE A CHANGE TODAY!

I cannot overstate the importance of reading God's Word—it
will literally bring you life spiritually and physically. Here are
some tips that will help you develop a habit of feeding your spirit
with the Word of God each day.

- **Decide to read your owner's manual now.** Make a
  commitment to God that you will read and heed His
  Word—not just in spiritual matters but in health
  matters as well.

- **Make a date.** Just as you write other commitments
  on your calendar or in your daily planner, schedule
  time to spend in God's Word. Is any appointment
  more important?

- **Tell your friends and family.** By sharing with
  others your intention to read and heed God's Word,
  you will hold yourself accountable (and so might
  they).

- **Find a Bible buddy.** Ask your spouse, neighbor,
  friend, sister, or brother to join you each day in
  reading the Word. If you can't meet face-to-face,
  touch base by phone or e-mail to share what you
  gleaned.

- **Keep a journal.** It doesn't have to be fancy. Write
  down the chapter and verses you read. Think about
  how those verses apply to your own situation and
  briefly record your thoughts.

Let's pray together.

> *God, You want me healthy. You want me well. Your words are life to me. They are medicine to all my flesh. I commit today to read and apply Your Word with active, living faith to my spirit, soul, and body. I am expecting and will experience a happy, healthier future. In Jesus's name, amen.*

I am going to make a change today. Here's how:

2   Relax in the Lord

*Come to Me, all you who labor and are heavy-laden and
overburdened, and I will cause you to rest. [I will ease and
relieve and refresh your souls.] Take My yoke upon you and
learn of Me, for I am gentle (meek) and humble (lowly) in
heart, and you will find rest (relief and ease and refreshment and recreation and blessed quiet) for your souls. For My
yoke is wholesome (useful, good—not harsh, hard, sharp, or
pressing, but comfortable, gracious, and pleasant), and My
burden is light and easy to be borne.*

—MATTHEW 11:28–30

S INCE I HAVE been teaching about healthy living, I've discovered ten practical keys to good health that God has given us in His Word. One of them is that we must *learn to relax.* This simple activity has profound effects on your mental, emotional, and physical condition.

Stress is arguably the number one enemy of your immune system. Stress sets the body up for all kinds of diseases—from diabetes to high blood pressure to gastrointestinal problems such as irritable bowel syndrome. It can also be linked to many life-threatening conditions, including heart disease, cancer, and kidney disease. Trying to treat an illness without addressing the stress causing it is like not seeing the forest for the trees!

Many times even the most conscientious health care providers fall into the trap of relieving only the symptoms of a disease instead of helping the patient resolve the underlying stressors causing it. In many cases the situation gets even more complicated when doctors prescribe pharmaceutical drugs that cover the symptoms instead of treating the root of the illness. As a result, the condition gets worse. I am sad to say that this is the rule, not the exception, in today's drug-oriented health care system.

Instead, try God-oriented health care. God knows how your body functions—after all, He made it! And we can get to know the mind of our Maker by reading our owner's manual, which is God's Word. As you follow God's manual, you will find that it comes with a guarantee. God gave this guarantee to mankind when He walked this earth as the man Jesus Christ.

We read this guarantee in John 10:10, where Jesus says He came so we could "have and enjoy life, and have it in abundance (to the full, till it overflows)." The Greek word translated "life" in this verse means "absolute fullness of life." It's a life without sickness, disease, or anything that can prevail against God's plan for you.

How do you discover this disease-free life? First, you learn to relax. Jesus said it best in Matthew 11:28–29, "Come to Me, all you who labor and are heavy-laden and overburdened, and I will cause you to rest. [I will ease and relieve and refresh your souls.] Take My yoke upon you and learn of Me, for I am gentle (meek) and humble (lowly) in heart, and you will find rest (relief and ease and refreshment and recreation and blessed quiet) for your souls."

There you go! The key to learning to relax is coming to Jesus, learning from Him, and doing things His way. Don't worry—His way is not the hard way. In fact, it is the easiest way. He guarantees it in verse 30: "For My yoke is easy and My burden is light" (NKJV).

MAKE A CHANGE TODAY!

Decades ago research found that practicing relaxation techniques can bring a host of health benefits, including:

- Strengthening the immune system
- Widening respiratory passages of people with asthma
- Reducing the need for insulin in people with diabetes
- Significantly relieving chronic pain
- Helping ward off disease by making people less susceptible to viruses
- Lowering blood pressure and cholesterol levels[1]

Here are three ways to relax during the workday. Find a quiet place where you can sit down comfortably and, if possible, not be disturbed.

1. **Become prayerfully aware**. Begin by closing your eyes and silently praising and thanking the Lord for your life. For example, repeat the phrases "Thank You, Lord, for my life" or "Praise You, Lord, for Your love." As you repeat these phrases silently, notice that your body and mind are relaxing. In your mind's eye imagine a peaceful, comfortable place. Breathe slowly and deeply. If you feel any tension in any body part, consciously let it go.

2. **Perform a muscle inventory**. Starting with your feet and working up, progressively tense and release each body part: calves, thighs, buttocks, abdomen, shoulders, arms, hands, and face. After releasing the muscle, release it a little bit more. Take five deep breaths in and out and repeat the tense-release progression one more time.

3. **Imagine the warm light of God's love**. Imagine a warm white light shining on the top of your head. Tell yourself that the light is relaxing all the muscles

of your head. Move the imaginary light to your jaw, throat, shoulders, arms, and hands. Feel the warmth and respond by loosening all tension. Let the light move to your abdomen, thighs, legs, feet, and toes. Then imagine your whole body bathed in the warm white light of God's love as you let go of any remaining tension.

Let's pray together.

Lord, I choose to discover and enjoy Your pathway to life and health by learning to relax according to Your holy Word. In Jesus's name, amen.

I am going to make a change today. Here's how:

3   Drink More Water

Now on the final and most important day of the Feast, Jesus stood, and He cried in a loud voice, If any man is thirsty, let him come to Me and drink! He who believes in Me [who cleaves to and trusts in and relies on Me] as the Scripture has said, From his innermost being shall flow [continuously] springs and rivers of living water.

—JOHN 7:37-38

DON'T HAVE TO tell you that you need water to live. But chances are you're not drinking enough. According to Pastor Stan Moore, author of *Living Well by Water*, most of us drink only two glasses of water a day—or less.[1] The US Geological Survey reports that the average person drinks up to four cups of water a day.[2] Either way, most people don't drink nearly enough water. God does not want you to get sick, but you must do your part and stay hydrated. Perhaps that's why He included more than seven hundred references to water in His Word.

Think of your body as a sponge. When a sponge is dried out, it's brittle, cracks easily, and is not much use for anything. Soldiers know how important water is. The three things they are taught to protect are their lives, their guns, and their canteens.

Have you ever worked out hard and gotten all hot and sweaty? Doesn't a cool glass of water taste good then? Well, water is that good for your body all the time, even when you haven't been working out.

You can stay alive for forty days without food—but only seven days without water. How much water should you drink each day? Divide your weight in pounds by two—that's how many ounces of water you need each day. To keep it simple, on average, people need eight to ten 8-ounce glasses of water. Eight glasses will keep you hydrated. Drinking ten helps you detoxify.

The earth is roughly three quarters water, and a healthy body is also made up mostly of water. Your vital organs are 70 percent to 90 percent water. A healthy brain is roughly 70 percent water, and blood is 83 percent water.[3] As is written in Leviticus 17:11, the life of the flesh is in the blood. In the Gospel of John alone Jesus talked about "living water" four times.

Make a Change Today!

Drinking two 8-ounce glasses of water before meals is not just good for your overall health, but it can also help you lose weight. A 2010 clinical trial found that over the course of twelve weeks, dieters who drank water before meals three times a day lost about five pounds more than dieters who did not increase their water intake.[4] Drinking water before meals fills the stomach so you eat less.

Another way to combat pounds is to drink water instead of soda pop or other sugary drinks. That includes artificially sweetened "diet" drinks, as these have been shown to increase appetite.[5]

A lot of people struggle to drink enough water every day, so here's a good way to get your eight to ten glasses. When you get up in the morning, drink two 8-ounce glasses of water. During the day say no to soda pop or sweetened drinks. Drink pure water instead. When you get home at the end of the day, sit down and enjoy a nice glass of water on ice or with a slice of lemon.

Keep your sponge—your body—moist, flexible, and healthy, not dry, brittle, and thirsty. Eight glasses a day will keep sickness—and unwanted weight—away!

Let's pray together.

> *Lord, I am a water drinker. I love to drink water. I will try to drink eight to ten glasses of water every day. In Jesus's name, amen.*

I am going to make a change today. Here's how:

4 Try the Genesis Diet

*Then the Lord God formed man from the dust of the ground
and breathed into his nostrils the breath or spirit of life, and
man became a living being.*

—GENESIS 2:7

YOU'VE HEARD IT said, "You are what you eat." As far as
your physical body is concerned, that's exactly true. Genesis 2:7 says God formed man from the dust of the ground.
In fact, the word *human* is from the Latin word *humus*, which
can be translated to mean earth. Mankind was made from the
humus—the dirt of the ground.

God breathed life into the nostrils of this *humus man*, and
he became a living being with a soul. The Targum, the Aramaic
translation-paraphrase of Scripture, says Adam became "another
speaking spirit."[1]

That's who you are—another speaking spirit, made in the
image of God. While you live on this earth, you have your own
"humus body," what I like to call your "earth suit." You get to stay
here only as long as your earth suit lasts. When your earth suit
wears out, you must and will leave this planet, though the real
you—your spirit—lives on in eternity.

This Genesis story brings up a divine principle: you must stay
connected to what you came from to stay strong. This is certainly true for your spirit man. You came from God's Spirit. To
stay strong spiritually you must stay in tune with God's Spirit.
You accomplish this by reading God's Word, talking with Him
in prayer, and thanking and praising Him for your life. Without
a constant spiritual connection, your spirit dries up.

This principle holds true for your physical body as well. To stay strong as God intended, you must stay connected to where your body came from—the dirt. How do you stay connected to the dirt? Through the foods you eat. This is how it works: the farmer plants a seed in the dirt. With proper sunlight and water the seed literally reorganizes the dirt it was sown in to form a plant. Then you come along and eat this reorganized dirt in the form of a plant. As you digest, absorb, and reorganize the dirt again, it becomes a part of your body.

Your physical body is nothing more than reorganized dirt! Without staying connected to this reorganized dirt we call plant food, our physical bodies can last only around forty to sixty days at the most. Many people could not stay alive for even thirty days without eating. This is how God set up your earthly existence.

Because God made food important, He also made sure to give you specific, insightful information in the first chapter of the Bible to guide your eating habits. I call it the Genesis diet. Your body is going to love it because it was specifically designed for you. Today let's agree to strive to understand and follow God's system of eating to obtain optimum health.

MAKE A CHANGE TODAY!

Seeds aren't just for planting. Genesis 1:12 says, "The earth brought forth vegetation, plants yielding seed after their kind, and trees bearing fruit with seed in them, after their kind; and God saw that it was good" (NAS). While fresh fruits and vegetables are indeed superior foods, remember to include seeds in your diet as well.

+ **Flaxseeds.** These contain high amounts of healthy, omega-3 fatty acids for heart health; lignans, which help ensure regularity; and mucilage, which increases the intestines' ability to absorb needed nutrients. Hide these seeds in oatmeal, sprinkle them lightly on salads, or bake them into muffins. Flaxseed oil can be mixed into salad dressings or beverages.[2]

+ **Sesame seeds.** Add a nutty crunch to stir-fry, salad dressings, and even peanut butter sandwiches by using sesame seeds. Rich in essential minerals, sesame seeds support heart and lung health, lower risks for osteoporosis, and may help reduce the pain of migraines and PMS.[3]

+ **Pumpkin seeds.** Like their little cousins sesame seeds, pumpkin seeds, also called pepitas, offer a wealth of beneficial minerals. They may also boost prostate health and lower cholesterol.[4]

+ **Sunflower seeds.** These are not just for the kids! A great source of vitamin E, sunflowers may help reduce asthma symptoms and relieve arthritis pain. They can also calm your nerves, lower risk for cancer, and help relieve menopausal hot flashes.[5]

+ **Cumin seeds.** Commonly used in Mexican, Middle Eastern, and Indian fare, cumin seeds can also add some spice to stir-fried, steamed, or grilled vegetables. An excellent source of iron, cumin aids digestion and may help prevent cancer.[6]

Eating a Genesis diet—the foods God designed your body to best digest—will pay off in the long run and put you on the road to longevity and lasting health.

Let's pray together.

> *Lord, You made me fearfully and wonderfully, and You want me to have a perfectly functioning body. I will feed my body according to Your instructions. I am Your child. I like good foods. Your foods are good foods. Therefore, I like Your foods. In Jesus's name, amen.*

I am going to make a change today. Here's how:

5   Get to Bed on Time

In peace I will both lie down and sleep, for You, Lord, alone make me dwell in safety and confident trust.

—Psalm 4:8

GET TO BED on time! Sounds simple enough, doesn't it? But for many it is one of the most difficult of God's health rules to follow. Not getting enough sleep for even two or three nights can cause your mental and physical abilities to severely deteriorate. Psalm 4:8 says, "I will both lie down in peace, and sleep; for you alone, O LORD, make me to dwell in safety" (NKJV).

God designed you to get a peaceful night's sleep. Think about it for a moment. Sleep is a rather strange occurrence. All day long you run full speed ahead, and then suddenly, after about sixteen hours, your brain and your body tell you, "We have to stop what we're doing and rest for the next eight hours!"

This happens every day of your life, 365 days a year! During sleep your brain continues to function but at a much different level. Bodily functions carry on but not in the same manner as when you are awake. Your body needs rest because rest brings restoration.

Your body literally needs a time-out to rebuild, restore, and replenish all of your body's various systems. Without this restoration you cannot fight off sickness and disease. Your body began that fight while you were still within your mother's womb, and you must continue that battle every single day of your life.

I like to compare the immune system to an army. Every day of your life enemy bacteria, viruses, and toxins invade your body. Your immune system has to be ready at all times to combat them. To maintain battle readiness, you must feed your troops, replenish their munitions, and let them rest. Your immune system needs the eight-hour interval you call sleep to recharge for another day on the front. Sleep is essential to your immune system's strength and survival. In other words, when you get enough sleep, you get sick less often.

The immune system isn't the only body system that relies on sleep to maintain healthy function. All of your vital organs require a daily tune-up—a tune-up that takes place only when you sleep. Your brain initiates the restoration phase during deep REM sleep. (REM stands for rapid eye movement.) Dreams occur during REM sleep. Without this level of sleep you put yourself at risk for various psychoses and emotional disorders.

Your musculoskeletal system demands rest times too. Without it your muscles become exhausted and cramp up. Your heart is a muscle. Every beat it makes and every breath you take depends on your having a good habit of regular, good sleep.

You can say no to sickness, heart disease, and mental and emotional problems by simply enjoying a good night's sleep. Thank God for the gift of sleep!

MAKE A CHANGE TODAY!

Do you know how much sleep you need? The National Sleep Foundation has determined the following sleep-need ranges for various age groups.

- Adults: seven to nine hours
- Teens: eight and a half to nine and a quarter hours
- Schoolchildren: ten to eleven hours
- Toddlers: twelve to fourteen hours

+ Infants: fourteen to fifteen hours
+ Newborns: twelve to eighteen hours[1]

Studies have found that when you don't get enough sleep, your productivity decreases, you have trouble remembering things, and you raise your risks for automobile accidents, gaining unhealthy weight, substance abuse, and developing heart problems, diabetes, depression.[2] Perhaps parents should be advising their teenagers to "Just go to sleep" rather than "Just say no!"

"There is strong evidence that sufficient shortening or disturbance of the sleep process compromises mood, performance and alertness and can result in injury or death," wrote sleep researchers Michael H. Bonnet and Donna L. Arand. "In this light, the most common-sense 'do no injury' medical advice would be to avoid sleep deprivation."[3]

Praise God that we can have restful sleep when we put our confidence in Him. It will do our bodies good!

Let's pray together.

> *Lord, I will both lie down in peace and sleep, for You alone, O Lord, make me to dwell in safety. I thank You that I am a great sleeper. Every night when I sleep, I thank You for yet another opportunity to make my sleep habits better and better. In Jesus's name, amen.*

I am going to make a change today. Here's how:

6 Begin to Exercise

For physical training is of some value (useful for a little), but godliness (spiritual training) is useful and of value in every-thing and in every way, for it holds promise for the present life and also for the life which is to come.

—1 TIMOTHY 4:8

TODAY I'D LIKE you to consider the importance of consistent exercise. Exercise is not something you *have* to do; it is something you *get* to do! The hardest part of exercising is deciding to start. Once you've made the decision to begin exercising, you will experience so many healthful and enjoyable benefits, you'll get hooked on it for life!

God created you to exercise—and He created exercise for you. That's what your body's owner's manual (the Bible) says. First Timothy 4:8 tells us, "Bodily exercise profits a little, but godliness [spiritual exercise] is profitable for all things" (NKJV). Because of that word *little* Christians often interpret this verse to mean that physical exercise is not important. This is not the true intention of the passage.

The original Greek translation of the phrase "profits little" is "profitable for a season." The season the Word refers to here is your season of physical life here on earth. Physical exercise is extremely profitable for you as long as you live in your physical body. Your longevity here on Planet Earth directly depends on how well you take care of your earth suit. When your body wears out—time's up!

Of course, your spirit lives on, leaving your old dead body behind. To be absent from the body is to be present with the

Lord! So what do we need to know about that spiritual exercise? Reading your Bible and praying is always a good daily workout, one that helps you to discover and walk in God's will.

Spiritual exercise will also profit you in the world to come. Even in your glorified body you'll need to stay connected to God. But you won't need to do sit-ups, push-ups, or daily cardio anymore! The physical laws of this planet that make exercise essential will no longer apply. Philippians 3:20–21 says, "For our citizenship is in heaven, from which we also eagerly wait for the Savior, the Lord Jesus Christ, who will transform our lowly body that it may be conformed to His glorious body" (NKJV). Hallelujah!

Until that day, the way to transform your earthly body is through consistent, moderate physical exercise. For the season you are on this earth, bodily exercise will profit you. Do you want to feel better, look better, and have more energy? Make the decision now to exercise.

Make a Change Today!

Have you started plenty of exercise programs only to drop out a few months or so down the road? Well, you're not alone. Researchers have found that half of us do just that. Why? Here's what the researchers discovered.

- ♦ **Poor self-image.** If you feel incompetent while exercising, you are less likely to start a fitness regimen and more likely to quit if you do begin one. Women with low self-worth are even less likely to continue an exercise regime.

- ♦ **Excess weight.** People with extra pounds have more trouble sticking with exercise programs.

+ **Unrealistic expectations.** People who set unrealistic strength-training or weight-loss goals are more likely to give up exercising.
+ **Practical barriers.** Many people simply don't have the time or place to exercise.[1]

Are any of these roadblocks to fitness standing in your way? Identifying the problem is the first step toward solving it. Remember, improving your fitness level may help you overcome your self-esteem and weight issues. The same researchers also identified what motivates people to stay with a program:

+ **Clear goals.** For example, those who aim to remain independent as they age are more likely to continue exercising.
+ **Positive reinforcement.** Those who ask family members and friends to encourage them in their exercise goals stand a better chance of success.
+ **Professional training.** Individuals who enlist a personal trainer or coach benefit from a program tailored to their needs.
+ **Exercising in groups.** The camaraderie and accountability of groups can do wonders for making you stick with a program. Researchers also found that watching other people exercise is great motivation.
+ **Being consistent.** Make an appointment with your body every day. You wouldn't skip a doctor's appointment, would you? Well, exercising can do more for your health than any number of doctors ever will. [2]

If you need to make exercising a priority, try some of the strategies above that have worked for others. Set clear goals for yourself, ask friends and family members to encourage you in your fitness goals, consider enlisting a personal trainer, and think about finding an exercise buddy or a group activity. Above all, make a daily appointment with your body. Committing to exercise consistently will profit you for the rest of your life.

Let's pray together.

> God, You made my body to benefit tremendously from exercise. You want me to exercise. I know You will help me to exercise consistently. From now on I commit to exercising regularly. I will not make excuses. In Jesus's name, amen.

I am going to make a change today. Here's how:

7   Calm Your Mind

*You will guard him and keep him in perfect and constant
peace whose mind [both its inclination and its character] is
stayed on You, because he commits himself to You, leans on
You, and hopes confidently in You.*

—Isaiah 26:3

I HAVE A FAVORITE health proverb. It's Proverbs 14:30, "A calm and undisturbed mind and heart are the life and health of the body, but envy, jealousy, and wrath are as rottenness to the bones."

The first few words of that proverb are loaded with so much insight into your health that I could teach an entire seminar on them. What does "a calm and undisturbed mind and heart" mean? And how do you obtain such calmness?

"A calm and undisturbed mind and heart" means having peace of mind and peace of soul. This state of quiet rest supports you regardless of circumstances.

Is such an inner calm truly possible, when life seems to bring some new problem every day? I don't pretend to know what you are going through, but I do know God. He promises in Hebrews 4:3 that when you believe, you enter into His rest. "Believe what?" you may ask. Believe what God's Word says about you.

For example, Philippians 4:19 says God will supply all of your needs. That promise can surely bring you peace of mind—if you believe it. Isaiah 26:3 specifically promises "perfect and constant peace" for those "whose mind [both its inclination and its character] is stayed" on God.

Not only does God's Word promise you perfect peace, but it

also promises that you can remain in that perfect peace as long as you keep your mind on God—on His plans, His promises, and His thoughts about you. Jeremiah 29:11 says God knows the plans He has for you, plans for peace and not evil.

In the original Hebrew the word translated "peace" in Jeremiah 29:11 is *shalom*. Shalom simply means "complete" or "whole." In other words, nothing missing and nothing broken. That is God's plan for you right now—that you would lack nothing, and nothing would be broken in your life. This includes your physical body and your soul—your mind, will, and emotions. Doesn't that promise give you great peace inside?

Now let's review Proverbs 14:30. What will having a calm and undisturbed mind and heart do for you? They are the life and health of your body. Why? Because what happens on the inside affects what happens on the outside.

Tell me what you're thinking about, and I'll tell you what you are. You will always proceed in the direction of your dominant thoughts. Proverbs 23:7 says as a man thinks in his heart, so is he. What has your heart been thinking about lately?

If you don't like what is going on in your physical body, you can change it. But that change is going to have to start with a change of thought. Decide today to have life and health in your body by actively keeping your mind on God. If you lean on Him, you will lack nothing, and nothing will be broken in your life.

MAKE A CHANGE TODAY!

According to biblical scholars, clasping your hands in prayer does more than signal that you are in conversation with the Lord. The common prayer gesture dates back before the time of Christ.

Some believe that when you bring your right and left hands together, you join the left and right hemispheres of your brain.

"Such a gesture is said to calm the mind," writes prayer blogger Babes Tan-Magkalas. "I find that I am able to focus more on God and concentrate better when I pray using the praying hands gesture. It's as if folding or clasping or drawing my hands together sends a signal to my mind to calm down."[1]

Is your mind racing ahead with worries about what might happen next or memories of yesterday's pain? Reclaim the calmness of being in the present moment by clasping your hands together and taking a moment to commune with God.

Let's pray together.

> God, You keep me in perfect peace because I keep my mind on Your promises. I declare that I have a calm, undisturbed mind and heart, which is life and health to my body. In Jesus's name, amen.

I am going to make a change today. Here's how:

8 Clean the Inside of Your Body

*And whoever gives to one of these little ones [in rank or influ-
ence] even a cup of cold water because he is My disciple,
surely I declare to you, he shall not lose his reward.*

—Matthew 10:42

ET'S TALK AGAIN about water. Do you remember the
story of the Samaritan woman in the fourth chapter of
the Gospel of John? As Jesus watched her draw water
from the well, He said to her, "Give Me a drink" (v. 7). God
Himself, when He walked as a man on earth, drank water.

I always encourage people to drink what they are mostly
made of, which is fresh, pure water. Your vital organs, skeletal
system, immune system, eyes, ears, brain, and each of your teeny,
tiny cells are composed of 75 percent to 80 percent water (if you
are healthy). You simply cannot enjoy optimal health if you are
dehydrated. Your body thirsts for water because water is such
an integral part of all its members—and all of its processes. Not
one cell can stay alive, let alone function, without adequate water.

You are only as healthy as your individual cells. Each cell is
like a tiny factory that takes in raw materials and transforms
them through millions of different chemical reactions. Nearly
all of these processes require water. Water keeps your cells alive,
and your cells keep you alive.

Each of these processes also produces waste that is poten-
tially toxic to your body. If your body does not properly eliminate these toxic wastes, you become unhealthy. Lack of adequate
water severely limits your body's ability to eliminate toxins.

You see, water is your body's most vital solvent. It is the fluid that carries all the vital elements—oxygen, hormones, and other chemical messengers—to each one of your cells. Another function of cells is communication. Without adequate water your cells are not able to communicate with one another properly. When this happens, your tissues and organs begin to malfunction. Disease takes root. A dehydrated body gets sick.

On the other hand, a hydrated body is a healthy body. The more you learn about water, the thirstier you'll get. The truth is that many people who think they are sick really aren't. They are just thirsty. Too many people are treating simple dehydration with over-the-counter and prescription medications. These medications leave even more toxins in the body, which require even more water if they are to be properly eliminated. I like to say that water is a natural medication with no side effects!

Your body literally cries out for water. Perhaps that's one reason Jesus said, "Whoever gives these little ones only a cup of cold water…shall by no means lose his reward" (Matt. 10:42, NKJV).

MAKE A CHANGE TODAY!

Dehydration can be dangerous, so please don't take it lightly. It's good for everyone to drink eight to ten glasses of water each day. But if you have any of the following risk factors listed by the Mayo Clinic website, you need to be even more vigilant about drinking enough water daily.

+ **Advanced age.** As you get older, your body has less ability to conserve water and doesn't always tell you when you're thirsty. If you live alone, you may even forget to drink water. Because your body does not respond to temperature changes as it did when you

were younger, dehydration can put you at higher
risk of heat stroke too. These issues can become
even more aggravated if you have diabetes, are experiencing menopausal hormone fluctuations, or are
taking certain prescription medications.

+ **Chronic illness**. Diabetes, kidney disease, alco-
holism, and adrenal gland disorders increase your risk
for dehydration.

+ **Colds, flu, and sore throat**. These conditions may
reduce your desire to drink water, which can lead
to dehydration. If you have a fever, you are at even
higher risk of becoming dehydrated.

+ **Strenuous exercise**. Whenever you exercise, you
need to replenish fluids, especially in hot and
humid weather. If you're training for a marathon,
mountain climbing, or participating in some other
high-intensity activity, you can actually lose more
water than you take in, resulting in dangerous dehydration over a period of time. Make sure you drink
enough water every day to replace what you may have
lost.

+ **Living in high altitudes**. If you spend your time
above 8,200 feet, your body tries to adjust by
increasing urination and speeding up breathing. Both
deplete your body of water. Drink more water on a
regular basis to offset this.

+ **Being out in hot, humid weather**. When the air
is hot and humid, your sweat can't evaporate so
your body heats up more quickly. Drink extra water
to combat this, especially if you are exercising or
engaging in other vigorous physical activity.[1]

Whether or not you are at greater risk of dehydration, commit today to drink an adequate amount of water. It's the only way to keep your body functioning as God intended.

Let's pray together.

> *I am Your child, Lord. I need water. Water is the drink You recommend, so I am a water drinker. I love to drink my eight glasses of water every day. In Jesus's name, amen.*

I am going to make a change today. Here's how:

9   Eat Bible Foods

*And God said, See, I have given you every plant yielding
seed that is on the face of all the land and every tree with
seed in its fruit; you shall have them for food.*

—Genesis 1:29

WE'VE ALREADY DISCUSSED the importance of staying
connected to the soil our physical bodies were formed
from. (See chapter 4, "Try the Genesis Diet.") You
accomplish this by eating God-made foods from the earth,
namely fruits, vegetables, and whole grains.

Your food choices have a tremendous impact on your health.
Good choices yield good health. Poor choices yield poor health.

God did not even let the first chapter of His Word go by
without giving us His good advice on how to eat. Bible scholars
often refer to the "law of first mention." The first time the Bible
mentions a specific subject, that scripture is giving divine revela-
tion and foundational wisdom into that topic.

Undoubtedly this is the case in Genesis 1:29, which tells
us, "Every plant yielding seed…and every tree with seed in its
fruit; you shall have them for food." What is this verse telling
us? Simply put, it is saying we should eat fruits, vegetables, and
whole grains. These are God-made foods. Real foods. Whole
foods. Complete foods. Not man-made foods. If you do not eat
God's real foods, you are going to get into real trouble.

Take a look at what else the Bible says about what you eat.
First Corinthians 10:31 says, "Therefore, whether you eat or
drink, or whatever you do, do all to the glory of God" (NKJV).

This verse says you can actually eat to the glory of God. It also implies that you can eat in a manner that does not glorify God.

Choosing to eat the way God wants you to is inarguably one of the best ways to get and stay healthy. Another verse makes an even stronger connection between good health and the foods we eat. Exodus 23:25 says, "So shall you serve the LORD your God, and He will bless your bread and your water. And I will take sickness away from the midst of you" (NKJV).

Imagine having sickness and disease taken away from you—simply because God's blessing is upon your food and water! This truth is so wonderful that I have taught it to my children. When we sit down to dinner, my children recite this verse as we pray over our food. I can think of few things that have greater influence over your health than your food choices.

Make a Change Today!

Bread is a staple of the standard American diet, but not all breads are created equal. Breads loaded with whole grains are a much healthier option. You can buy Ezekiel bread, which is made from sprouted grains and typically does not contain flour, at large supermarkets and health food stores. But if you want to be adventurous, you can try my version of Ezekiel bread. It uses many of the healthy ingredients found in Ezekiel 4:9, but unlike traditional Ezekiel bread, it doesn't require you to sprout and grind your own grains. Plan on it taking about three hours, which includes the time it takes for the bread to rise.

Dr. Don's Ezekiel Bread

8 cups 100 percent whole-wheat flour or gluten-free all purpose flour

4 cups barley flour

½ cup millet flour

¼ cup rye flour

2 cups lentils, cooked and mashed

1½ cups water

1 Tbsp. salt

4–6 Tbsp. olive oil

2 packets of yeast

½ cup warm water

1 Tbsp. honey

Directions:

1. Preheat oven to 375 degrees.

2. Dissolve yeast in the warm water. Let stand for ten minutes.

3. Combine all flours.

4. Mix lentils, oil, and a little water (from the 1½ cups) in blender or food processor. Pour mixture in large mixing bowl and combine with remaining water.

5. Stir in 2 cups of flour mixture; then mix in yeast.

6. Stir in salt and remaining flour.

7. Knead dough on floured breadboard until smooth.

8. Place dough in oiled bowl and let rise until it has doubled in bulk.

9. Knead dough again. Shape into four loaves. Place loaves in four greased loaf pans. Let rise again until loaves have doubled in bulk.

10. Bake for 45 minutes to 1 hour.

Let's pray together.

Heavenly Father, I thank You for blessing my food and water and for taking sickness and disease from my midst. Help me to make food choices that are better for me and that glorify You. In Jesus's name, amen.

I am going to make a change today. Here's how:

10 Sleep Better and Live More Productively

It is vain for you to rise up early, to take rest late, to eat the bread of [anxious] toil—for He gives [blessings] to His beloved in sleep.

—Psalm 127:2

WE'VE ALREADY TALKED about the importance of sleep, but this topic is so crucial I need to spend some more time on the significance of having good sleep habits. How much sleep you get every night affects many areas of your life—some may surprise you.

In chapter 5, "Go to Bed on Time" I encouraged you to claim the blessing of Psalm 4.8, "I will both lie down in peace, and sleep; for You alone, O LORD, make me dwell in safety" (NKJV). The problem is if you are not going to bed on time, you cannot possibly enjoy this luxury from God, the luxury of being able to lie down in peace and sleep.

How much sleep is enough? People's sleep needs vary; no magical number of hours applies to everyone. While some people may seem to function fairly well on as little as five hours of sleep a night, new research has found that at least seven to nine hours are required.

Some people need ten hours of sleep—and some even more than that. Is that too much? For most people, getting too much sleep is not a problem. However, if you think you are sleeping too much, you might want to investigate underlying physical or emotional issues that may be making you drowsy or lethargic.

If you are like millions of Americans, you may believe that cutting back on the time you spend sleeping will help you get more done in a day. Actually, sleep studies have proven that this fails. Skimping on sleep reduces your performance on the job and in the home. When you deprive yourself of sleep, you are less creative and less productive.

Dr. Richard Bootzin, professor of psychology and director of the insomnia clinic at the University of Arizona Sleep Disorder Center, has done long-term research on sleep. He found that people who get seven to eight hours of sleep every night not only live longer but also are healthier and happier than those who get less sleep.[1]

God shared the same information with His people thousands of years ago. Psalm 127:2 tells us, "It is vain for you to rise up early, to sit up late, to eat the bread of sorrows; for so He gives His beloved sleep" (NKJV).

What a great promise! Why not take advantage of it? By the way, other studies have determined that the best hours for healthy, restful sleep are between 10:00 p.m. and 2:00 a.m. Some researchers believe that every hour of sleep during these hours can equal up to two hours of sleep outside of them. Maybe that's why God created darkness every night.

Take steps to improve your sleeping habits. You'll live longer, be healthier, and feel happier!

MAKE A CHANGE TODAY!

Insomnia is a serious health issue, one that leads many to rely on prescription sleeping pills to get to sleep every night. The trouble is, studies have shown that sleeping pills don't really work. "Sleeping pills [are] hazardous to your health," says Dr. Daniel Kripke, a leading sleep researcher from the University of California San Diego. "People who take [them] die sooner than people who don't....Sleeping pill effects are just the opposite of what people hope."[2]

A National Institutes of Health study found that people taking sleeping pills get only an extra eleven minutes of sleep a night. Why do people keep taking sleeping pills? They induce anterograde amnesia. When people get up in the morning, they don't remember that they couldn't get to sleep the night before.[3]

Speaking of medications and insomnia, some prescription and over-the-counter drugs used to treat the following conditions can also prevent you from getting a good night's sleep:

+ Colds and allergies
+ High blood pressure
+ Heart disease
+ Thyroid disease
+ Birth control
+ Asthma
+ Pain medications
+ Depression (especially SSRI antidepressants)[4]

Instead of trying to get by on a few hours of sleep each night or taking prescription medication to help you sleep, try going to bed early enough to get seven to nine hours of sleep. Choose to unplug from whatever else is vying for your attention—you'll get more done in the end if you do. And if you have trouble falling asleep, spend some time praying, reading God's Word, or listening to soft praise and worship music. You'll find peace in God's presence and, as a result, a good night's sleep.

Let's pray together.

> *Lord, help me to get to bed on time. Your Word says You give Your beloved sleep—and that's me! So I declare today that I am a great sleeper, in Jesus's name, amen.*

I am going to make a change today. Here's how:

11 Watch Your Words

Death and life are in the power of the tongue, and they who indulge in it shall eat the fruit of it [for death or life].

—PROVERBS 18:21

MANY PEOPLE WOULD be surprised to know where the Bible says the power of life and death is found. Proverbs 18:21 says death and life are in the power of the tongue. That's right—a pathway to health or destruction lies right under your nose.

Our tongues enable us to swallow—and we certainly know that there is a strong relationship between our food and drink choices and the health we enjoy. We know the saying, "you are what you eat," but did you know you also "eat" your words?

Read the rest of Proverbs 18:21: "Death and life are in the power of the tongue, *and they who indulge in it shall eat the fruit of it* [for death or life]" (emphasis added). That means the words you choose to speak will literally yield fruit in your life.

Let me give you another biblical example of the power of words. The third chapter of James compares the tongue with a bit in a horse's mouth—a tiny device that turns the horse's whole body—and with the small rudder of a huge ship. Although it seems almost insignificant, the rudder determines where the ship will go.

James 3:6 says, "The tongue is so set among our members that it defiles the whole body" (NKJV). In other words, as insignificant as they may seem, the tongue and the words you use it to speak control your entire body. Perhaps that's why Ephesians 4:29 says to "let no corrupt word proceed out of your mouth" (NKJV).

It may surprise you, but your body obeys your words. That's right—your immune system is listening to what you say. You can choose to speak words of life over your body—that it will align with God's design for it. If you declare the truth of God's Word—that it is God's will that you be in good health—those words will yield good fruit in your life.

From my studies I've learned that the speech center of your brain takes precedence over all other areas of your brain, including the central nervous system, which controls your whole body.

In Matthew 12:37 Jesus went so far as to say your words determine your destiny. You can decide right now to let the power of your tongue work toward building yourself a healthy future by choosing to speak only words of life.

Make a Change Today!

"Sticks and stones may break my bones, but words will never hurt me." Do you remember chanting that childhood epitaph when some bully attacked you verbally? You knew the bully's words were hurting you, even though you told yourself they weren't. Well, guess what? Researchers agree—words do hurt.

A recent Harvard Medical School study found that children who suffered verbal abuse from their peers experienced physical damage to their developing brains. Specifically, the connections between their brains' right and left hemispheres did not develop normally. These children grew up to experience more depression, anxiety, and hostility, and even had more incidence of substance abuse.[1]

I bet you know which age group was the most vulnerable—that's right, middle schoolers. Cruel words do far more than hurt feelings. They actually cause the brain to create neurotoxins. Even if you eat only organic foods, drink pure water, and live where the air is clean, you can poison those around you when you make hurtful remarks.

What about those silent statements you constantly make to yourself—those self-condemning comments about not being worthy, beautiful, successful, or smart? Those can also poison the mind. When you catch yourself inflicting verbal self-abuse, stop immediately and remember Philippians 4:8: "Whatever is true, whatever is honorable, whatever is right, whatever is pure, whatever is lovely, whatever is of good repute, if there is any excellence and if anything worthy of praise, dwell on these things" (NAS). Then retract the abusive self-talk and begin to speak God's truth to yourself—no matter how awkward it may feel at first. Tell yourself:

- I am fearfully and wonderfully made (Ps. 139:14).
- I am forgiven (Col. 1:14).
- I am precious to God (Isa. 43:4).
- I am more than a conqueror (Rom. 8:37).
- God loves me (John 15:13; 16:27; Rom. 5:8; Eph. 3:17–19).
- I am valuable (1 Cor. 6:20).
- I have a sound mind (2 Tim. 1:7).
- "I can do all things through Christ who strengthens me" (Phil. 4:13, NKJV)

Repeat this process as often as necessary until the truth of what God thinks about you crowds out the abusive lies of the enemy. Choose to speak life—to yourself and others—and impart health to your body!

Let's pray together.

> *Lord, I choose right now to speak only words of life. From now on I'll say Your words, which are life and health to my body. By Your words I was healed. You have put before me life and death; therefore, I choose life—words of life to keep my body strong and healthy. In Jesus's name, amen.*

I am going to make a change today. Here's how:

12 Let Go of Envy, Jealousy, and Anger

A calm and undisturbed mind and heart are the life and health of the body, but envy, jealousy, and wrath are like rottenness of the bones.

—PROVERBS 14:30

ET'S GO BACK to my favorite health proverb and look into the rest of that scripture. Proverbs 14:30 says envy, jealousy, and anger rot the bones. This is one of the subtlest yet most common ways the enemy tries to steal our health.

Did you know that your bone marrow manufactures the cells of your immune system? God designed each of us with an automatic health-maintenance system we call the immune system. The immune system guards us against sickness at all times.

When bacteria, a fungus, virus, or parasite attacks your body, your immune system goes into action against the invasion. Your very own internal army begins manufacturing and releasing chemicals that destroy the unwanted intruders.

In some cases special antibodies surround the infectious agent and help usher it out of your body. This is why you don't get sick every time you are exposed to these potential disease-causing entities. This is a very good mechanism, since you're exposed to these sorts of pathogens all the time. You're not sick all the time thanks to your immune system—as long as it functions the way God designed it.

Now remember what Proverbs 14:30 said about your bones, the place in your body that manufactures your immune system. Envy, jealousy, and anger rot your bones. Rotten bones mean rotten bone marrow—and rotten bone marrow means a rotten immune system. In other words, envy, jealousy, and anger set you up for disease! These negative, fear-based emotions are among the most potent stressors your body deals with. And today's medical science has proven time and again that stress is the number one enemy of your immune system.

For example, when you get angry, your blood pressure rises, respiration increases, and nutritional demands and heart rate can skyrocket. Your body goes into survival mode, pumping most of your blood to your muscles. During this state of high alert your immune system is temporarily neglected. Perhaps that is why the Bible says not to let the sun go down on your anger (Eph. 4:26).

You need to resolve these negative emotions. When you let them dominate your life, you weaken your immune system. Make a decision right now to not let negative emotions destroy your ability to stay strong against sickness and disease. You can strengthen your immune system by praying today to receive God's forgiveness—and by forgiving others.

MAKE A CHANGE TODAY!

Are you jealous? Most of us have experienced that feeling at least once in our lives. While jealousy seldom improves a relationship, it does harm the person experiencing that emotion. Stress relief expert Lauren E. Miller found that jealousy-induced stress can lead to serious illness, even cancer. She says, "There are many emotions that course through your body during the day that can rapidly increase the stress hormone along with blood pressure in your body, jealousy being one of them."[1]

Harvard Medical School research has shown that 80 percent of disease is stress-related.[2] Jealousy is a high-stress condition. Why is it so stressful? Because like a sinus toothache, jealousy strikes a nerve at our very core: the feeling that we are not good enough, unworthy, or a failure.

God's solution to jealousy is Ephesians 1:6, "To the praise of the glory of His grace, by which He made us accepted in the Beloved" (NKJV). God accepts you, and this reflects your true value. It makes no sense to compare yourself with anyone else. That you are "accepted in the Beloved" means you are loved. Focus your attention on God's love for you, not on how you compare with someone else.

Let's pray together.

> *Dear Lord, I resist envy, jealousy, and anger and refuse to allow them to dominate my emotions. I have a calm and undisturbed mind and heart, and these are life and health to my body. In Jesus's name, amen.*

I am going to make a change today. Here's how:

13 Eat God's Perfect Food

You shall serve the Lord your God; He shall bless your bread and water, and I will take sickness from your midst. None shall lose her young by miscarriage or be barren in your land; I will fulfill the number of your days.

—Exodus 23:25–26

ET'S TALK MORE about Bible foods. But first let me give you a little quiz. What well-known Bible food has been shown to help your body lower LDL (bad cholesterol), fight viral infections, help stabilize blood sugar, decrease appetite, regulate bowel function, prevent tooth decay, and even fortify your body's efforts to decrease cancer cell growth? I'll give you the answer at the end of this teaching, but I'm sure you'll be adding a lot more of this whole food to your diet.

As I explained before, there is a strong correlation between the food we eat and our health. Exodus 23:25 says God will bless our food and water and take sickness and disease from our midst. Let's not stop there. The very next verse promises even more long-term health if we choose God-blessed foods. Verse 26 says, "No one shall suffer miscarriage or be barren in your land; I will fulfill the number of your days" (NKJV).

Remember Genesis 6:3? "And the LORD said, 'My Spirit shall not strive with man forever, for he is indeed flesh; yet his days shall be one hundred and twenty years'" (NKJV). Did you catch that? You can live to one hundred twenty. But I know that will not happen unless God's blessing is upon the foods you choose.

Living to one hundred twenty may not seem all that attractive if you anticipate being sickly, weak, and unable to function.

But look at Moses. He lived to be one hundred twenty. When the number of his days was fulfilled, God told him to climb a mountain and die. That takes a lot of stamina for a twenty-year-old, let alone someone who is one hundred twenty.

The Bible says Moses's strength was not lost at one hundred twenty; even his eyesight was still good. How can this be? Moses followed God's dietary laws. In fact, God revealed those laws through Moses in Leviticus 11 as well as in the Genesis diet we've been talking about. God's plan for you is to live long and strong by eating His chosen foods.

Another striking example of how diet is related to health is found in the first chapter of Daniel. Here Daniel and three other young Hebrew men don't want to defile themselves with the food given to the Babylonians. So they ask to be given only pulse and water. Pulse is the Hebrew word *zara*, and it means something sown or planted in the ground and grown.

Once again we are back to the Genesis diet of fruits, vegetables, and whole grains. After only ten days the Hebrew youth looked healthier and had a better countenance than those who ate the Babylonian fare—and as a bonus God made them ten times wiser! God-made foods make a difference.

Now can you guess which food helps lower LDL and fights infections, and cancer while stabilizing blood sugar, decreasing appetite, and improving bowel function? It's what may be God's greatest fruit—the apple. I guess an apple a day really can help keep the doctor away. Maybe two can keep him away twice as long.

MAKE A CHANGE TODAY!

It's more than just a catchy phrase: an apple a day really will make a difference in your overall health. Here are seven ways to consume one apple each day.

1. Thinly sliced on top of a whole-grain pancake
2. Wedged and topped with peanut butter
3. Diced onto a salad
4. Chopped, tossed with cinnamon, and mixed into plain yogurt
5. Grated and mixed into oatmeal
6. Blended into an apple-banana smoothie
7. Grated into coleslaw or cooked cabbage

Let's pray together.

> *God, I am Your child. I like good foods. Your foods are good foods, so I like Your foods. I think I'll have an apple right now. In Jesus's name, amen.*

I am going to make a change today. Here's how:

14 Live Lean

So then, whether you eat or drink, or whatever you may do,
do all for the honor and glory of God.

—1 CORINTHIANS 10:31

WE KNOW OBESITY is a major health problem in our society. I hesitate to call it a disease because it's really a disorder of civilization. The standard American diet (SAD) offers so many wrong choices that are so easy to make. But in the long run you don't pay the price for good health habits; you pay the price for poor ones.

Achieving and maintaining your ideal weight is certainly one of the most essential steps you can take to improve your health. When we are trying to lose weight, we are really trying to lose fat, not lean muscle mass. So I use the pneumonic L-E-A-N to outline four simple tips for shedding those unwanted pounds.

L is for *liquids*. In this case, once again, the champion is good old water. With no calories, water is a great appetite suppressant, as it literally fills your stomach, leaving less room for higher calorie foods. I recommend two large glasses of water before meals. This one decision, when done consistently, can lead to significant weight loss all by itself.

E, as you might guess, is for *exercise*, which is not important for its calorie-burning ability alone. Exercise builds lean muscle mass. A pound of fat burns only a couple of calories in a day whereas a pound of muscle can burn up to fifty calories per day just because it's there.[1] The muscle you build literally becomes a calorie-burning machine. Because muscle has less volume than fat, you may see changes in your shape before experiencing overall

48

weight loss. By increasing your calorie-burning, lean muscle mass, you also are able to eat more without gaining weight.

A is for *avoiding* high-fat and sweet foods such as fried or junk foods. These foods are loaded with calories but lack nutrients. All they add to your life is pounds. *A* is also for *adding* fiber, especially in the form of vegetables. High-fiber foods not only help sweep away bad fats and toxins but also keep your bowels eliminating properly.

N is for *never* skipping meals and for *nibbling* on raw vegetables between meals. This will keep your metabolism burning all the time.

MAKE A CHANGE TODAY!

Are your kids overweight? Then it's time to do an extreme makeover on your pantry. A Pennsylvania State University study found that simply serving a smaller main dish portion encourages kids to eat more healthy sides such as vegetables and fruit. This can help your children lose unhealthy fat.[2] Deep-six the soda pop, white-flour pastas and crackers, store-bought cookies, sweet treats, chips, and chemical-laden convenience foods.

There other ways you can help your children slim down. For starters, turn off the TV, hide the video gaming system on the top shelf of a dark closet, and restrict computer time to homework use. Second, eliminate fast food. Give your family the wonderful opportunity to eat foods made from scratch in your own kitchen. What a blessing! Keep it simple. After all, raw fruits and vegetables are easy to prepare, and they are what you need most. Give your whole family a new nutritious start on wellness by adopting a LEAN lifestyle.

Let's pray together.

> *Lord, my liquid is water. I love to drink water. I am an
> exerciser, and I avoid junk foods and fat. I never skip
> meals and have a great metabolism. I'm on my way to
> my ideal weight. My body is a lean, clean, calorie-burning
> machine! In Jesus' name, amen.*

I am going to make a change today. Here's how:

15 Eat a Healthy Breakfast

*Who forbid people to marry and [teach them] to abstain from
[certain kinds of] foods which God created to be received
with thanksgiving by those who believe and have [an increas-
ingly clear] knowledge of the truth.*

—1 TIMOTHY 4:3

WE ALL HAVE a morning routine, but here is a healthy
way to start your day. Enjoy a good breakfast. The
way you start your day has an enormous effect on
how your body performs all day long, especially when it comes
to metabolism. Metabolism is simply the rate at which you burn
calories. Do you want your body to be a lean, clean, calorie-
burning machine? Then you must eat a healthy breakfast *every
day*.

Eating a healthy breakfast lets your body know it can keep
the fires of your metabolism burning because the fuel it needs—
food—is being supplied. In other words, eating a healthy breakfast turns the calorie-burning switch "on" and keeps it there all
day. If you skip breakfast, your body thinks it's in a starvation
situation and goes into survival mode. So it reduces metabolism
to conserve fuel and energy. This is why those who skip breakfast feel tired all day long instead of full of energy to perform
the day's tasks.

When the breakfast skipper also misses lunch, the problem is
magnified. When he or she finally eats late in the day or, worse
yet, just before bedtime, the body goes into storage mode, antici-
pating another day of insufficient fuel. All of this adds up to

excessive binge-type eating, fat accumulation, and suppressed metabolism.

Eating a healthy breakfast sets up your body to function well all day, but not all breakfasts are created equal. What should you eat? Try selecting at least two God-made foods (fruits, vegetables, or whole grains). For example, you can eat an apple, orange, or grapes with a piece of whole-grain toast. Or you can have some oatmeal with bananas, or a multi-grain cereal with skim milk or soymilk and a glass of fruit or vegetable juice. (If the juice is from concentrate, however, you'd be better off eating the whole fruit or vegetable.)

If you've never tried vegetables for breakfast, you will be surprised by how satisfying and filling the fiber in carrots or celery is first thing in the morning. These high-fiber foods really wake up the body and your metabolism—and slowly release energy to your body all morning long.

Since protein helps the brain wake up and stay alert, nuts and seeds, especially almonds and sunflower seeds, can be a great whole-grain choice. Some prefer to make a protein shake for breakfast, which is a great choice as long as it doesn't contain too much sugar. Blending in whole fruits is a good way to sweeten your shake without adding refined sugar.

What about good old-fashioned eggs and toast? There's nothing wrong with that combination. Just make sure the toast is whole grain and that you also drink a small glass of "not from concentrate" juice. Eggs, by the way, are a God-made food and a great way to begin your day with protein.

Don't forget to start your day with a couple of glasses of water. It will start to fill you up with no calories so you're not tempted to overeat these great breakfast foods.

Make a Change Today!

I know for a lot of people, there's barely enough time to get ready in the morning, much less eat breakfast. If that is the case for you, I'd encourage you to get up a little earlier if at all possible. Eating breakfast is that important. You can also eat a healthy breakfast on the go. Here are a few grab-and-go options:

- **Peanut butter (hold the jelly).** Spread that whole-wheat bagel, waffle, or pancake with protein-rich peanut butter instead of sugary jelly or syrup. Two tablespoons of peanut butter feeds you eight grams of protein as well as niacin, vitamin E, iron, riboflavin, and dietary fiber. Plus, there's no drip and no mess on your commute.

- **Fruit with cheese and nuts.** Keep a bowl of in-season fruit in your fridge or on your table. Grab a piece to go along with a sandwich bag full of cheese cubes and walnuts.

- **Frozen berry shake.** Drop a handful of frozen fruit into your blender—strawberries, cherries, blueberries, or peaches. Add a half-cup of plain yogurt and a half-cup of fat-free milk, and blend until fruity smooth.

- **Cereal parfait.** Layer your favorite whole-grain cereal flakes, raisins, walnut pieces, berries, and plain organic yogurt in a large to-go cup. Feel free to be creative and add other ingredients, such as coconut flakes, sunflower seeds, dried cranberries, or cherries.

Let's pray together.

> *Lord, I start my day the right way with God-made foods. I have a great metabolism and energy all day long. In Jesus's name, amen.*

I am going to make a change today. Here's how:

16 Think Well and Be Well

*Brethren, whatever is true, whatever is worthy of reverence
and is honorable and seemly, whatever is just, whatever is
pure, whatever is lovely and lovable, whatever is kind and
winsome and gracious, if there is any virtue and excellence,
if there is anything worthy of praise, think on and weigh and
take account of these things [fix your minds on them].*

—PHILIPPIANS 4:8

WHAT ACTIVITY WILL you spend more time doing
through the course of your life than any other—more
than eating, sleeping, or working? God's Word gives
a specific prescription for how to perform this important activity,
and it has a major impact on your health. What activity am I
referring to? It's *thinking.*

You're always thinking, whether about good things or bad,
true ones or false. Your thoughts can lead to positive or negative emotions; it can even cause pain. So what does God say
you should spend your time thinking about? "Whatever is true,
worthy of reverence and is honorable and seemly, whatever is
just, whatever is pure, whatever is lovely and lovable, whatever
is kind and winsome and gracious" (Phil. 4:8). Your thoughts
should meet all of those criteria; what you think about needs to
be more than just true.

Taking control of your thought life, with the help of the
Holy Spirit, will change your entire life because it will cause
you to make better decisions. As a result, your present and your
future will become much more positive. Most of the things you
worry about never even happen. Worry wastes your precious

thoughts—and it's a sin, because Jesus said in Luke 12:22–26, "Do not worry" (NKJV, see also Phil. 4:6). Worry is an expectation of the worst. It causes some of the worst kind of stress—and stress is the foremost enemy of your immune system.

When we choose to think as God instructs us to in Philippians 4:8, we reap the benefit of verse 9: "The God of peace (of untroubled, undisturbed well-being) will be with you." And, as we learned in Proverbs 14:30, "a calm and undisturbed mind and heart are the life and health of the body." Peace, life, and health! Sure sounds good, doesn't it?

MAKE A CHANGE TODAY!

When you worry, you stir up negative emotions—sadness, fear, and even anger. Researchers at the University of Wisconsin have found that activating brain regions associated with negative emotions weakened people's immune response to a flu vaccine. The researchers documented that negative emotions caused greater electrical activity in the right prefrontal cortex of the brain and led to a weaker immune response as long as six months later when they measured subjects for antibodies after they had received flu shots. Greater electrical activity in the left prefrontal cortex of the brain indicates a stronger immune response.[1]

Anger, fear, and sadness were three emotions that stimulated the right prefrontal cortex activity. Positive feelings such as enthusiasm and happiness stimulated the left prefrontal cortex. "[This is] some of the best evidence we've seen to date," says Dr. Janice Kiecolt-Glaser, a stress and immunity expert from Ohio State University College of Medicine. "They [emotions] have a very nice link to what happens if you meet a bacterium or a virus in real life."[2]

Decide today to let your thinking work *for* your good health instead of against it. Don't blindly accept whatever comes into your mind. Choose to think on things that bring God praise.

Let's pray together.

> *Lord, help me to spend my time thinking about only what-*
> *ever things are true, just, honest, pure, lovely, and of a good*
> *report. My thought life is blessed because I choose to think*
> *Your way. In Jesus's name, amen.*

I am going to make a change today. Here's how:

17 Eat Foods Your Heart Loves

Who satisfies your mouth [your necessity and desire at your personal age and situation] with good so that your youth, renewed, is like the eagle's [strong, overcoming, soaring]!

—PSALM 103:5

L ET'S TALK ABOUT how to have a healthy heart. This relatively small muscle pumps blood every second of every hour of every day—and if you want to stay alive, you'd better make sure it keeps pumping! The cardiovascular system is obviously one of the most vital, but it is also the most common organ system to be attacked by disease. Improper diet, poor lifestyle habits, and stress all have a major negative impact on your heart and will cut years off your life. How can you avoid this? By keeping your heart healthy.

I've developed an acronym from the letters of the word H-E-A-R-T that provides guidelines for giving this miraculous organ everything it needs for you to live long and strong. In today's tip, we'll focus on the first principle: *H* is for *healthy* foods and nutrients.

Your heart may be the most metabolically active tissue in your body. It requires a constant and immediate supply of vitamins and minerals, which are quickly consumed every time your heart muscle contracts. It makes sense that we should feed our hearts the vitamins and minerals it needs to function at its best. But which foods will keep your heart strong and your blood vessels clean? Which type of diet will help you best avoid a buildup of fat and cholesterol that can lead to heart attack, high blood pressure, or even a stroke?

The clear standout is the Mediterranean diet. This isn't a diet in the popular sense. Its aim isn't simply to help you lose weight. A Mediterranean diet draws from the eating habits of those in Mediterranean nations who eat an abundance of heart-healthy carbohydrates.

Good carbohydrates such as whole grains, breads, cereals, and pasta release energy slowly to the body. These foods—such as wheat, oats, rye, and brown rice—are loaded with fiber for cleaning out bad fats and detoxifying the body. They also are an abundant source of minerals, especially calcium and magnesium, which are absolutely essential for every heartbeat.

The next most common component of this heart-smart diet is fruits, vegetables, nuts, and beans. In general, the deeper the color of the fruit or vegetable, the more nutrients it contains. The healthiest nut is the almond. I recommend eating five to ten raw almonds a day as an excellent snack between meals. Beans of any kind are loaded with fiber as well as vitamins and minerals.

Another Mediterranean favorite is olive oil, which can be used instead of unhealthy margarine and high-fat butter and shortening. The heart-smart Mediterranean diet also includes moderate amounts of fish and eggs and small amounts of other meats and dairy products.

In the next tip I will explain the other components of the H-E-A-R-T acronym. But for now, remember that simple, God-made foods are the champions of a strong heart! Decide today to eat for longevity.

Make a Change Today!

Lifestyle changes begin with small choices. Instead of a traditional hamburger, why not try a heart-healthy bean burger? It's loaded with flavor and the nutrients your heart needs. And it's not loaded with the bad fats that can clog your arteries. My bean burger recipe is simple—and delicious.

Heart-Healthy Bean Burgers

1 (20-ounce) can black or adzuki beans, rinsed and drained

¼ cup yellow onion, diced

¼ cup red bell pepper, diced

½ tsp. ground cayenne pepper

1 egg

1 cup seasoned whole-grain breadcrumbs

2 Tbsp. fresh chopped cilantro

2 Tbsp. olive oil (optional)

Directions:

1. Preheat oven to 350 degrees. Use oil to grease baking pan.

2. Mash beans in a bowl. Add onion, bell pepper, cayenne pepper, egg, breadcrumbs, and cilantro. Blend well.

3. Form into six patties and place on baking pan.

4. Bake for ten minutes or fry the patties in olive oil over medium heat.

5. Serve on whole-grain buns with your favorite condiments and lettuce, tomato, and sliced onion, if desired.

Cooking from scratch is one of the best ways to ensure the foods you are eating are truly God-made—and it's more cost-effective if you're on a budget. There are many specialty "health" foods that can be great nutritionally, but they sometimes cost a lot. Whole, God-made foods may cost a bit more too, especially if you're used to buying heavily processed convenience foods. But bear in mind that the price of heart disease is even higher.

Let's pray together.

> *Lord, I choose to feed my heart the nutrients it needs by eating whole grains and fruits and vegetables. I include olive oil in my diet and select almonds and beans when I have a choice. My heart stays strong because I feed it properly. In Jesus's name, amen.*

I am going to make a change today. Here's how:

18 Enjoy a Heart-Healthy Lifestyle

Who satisfies your mouth [your necessity and desire at your
personal age and situation] with good so that your youth,
renewed, is like the eagle's [strong, overcoming, soaring]!

—PSALM 103:5

NOW THAT WE'VE examined the *H* in the H-E-A-R-T
acronym (eating *healthy* foods and nutrients), let's take
a look at what the rest of the letters represent.

E is for *exercise*! Consistent, moderate exercise is one of the
best ways to keep off those unwanted pounds, which require
miles of extra blood vessels and make your heart work so much
harder. People who exercise have slower heart rates, usually
below seventy-two beats per minute. Why? Because a heart
muscle that is in shape is much stronger and doesn't have to
beat as much to do the job. Hearts that are stronger last longer.
Exercise builds strong hearts.

Aerobic exercise is the most beneficial. This includes brisk
walking, jogging, dancing—basically anything that increases
your breathing rate and the blood's oxygen-carrying capacity,
making it easier for your heart to do its job.

Exercise also lowers blood pressure as well as bad cholesterol
(LDL) and fats in your blood. It increases your heart's collat-
eral circulation for a kind of "natural bypass" effect and increases
good cholesterol (HDL). If you don't know where to start with
an exercise program, I recommend thirty to forty minutes of
brisk walking three to five days a week.

A is for *antioxidants*! These fight free-radical damage that ages
the cardiovascular system. They include the ACES—vitamins

A, C, and E, and the trace mineral selenium, which are all found in the heart-smart fruits, vegetables, and whole grains mentioned previously. I also strongly recommend a daily multivitamin-minerals supplement to cover all the bases. It's a very inexpensive life insurance program for your heart.

R is for *restrict!* Restrict excess fats, especially saturated fats from animal sources and fried foods. Restrict simple sugars too—those found in junk and processed foods. This will help you keep your cardiovascular system lean and working well.

T is for *temperance.* Practice self-control and moderation in all things. When it comes to emotions, remember that a calm and undisturbed mind is the life and health of the body. In Luke 21:26 Jesus said men's hearts would fail them because of fear. But we know God hasn't given us a spirit of fear, but one of "power and of love...and discipline and self-control" (2 Tim. 1:7).

Make a Change Today!

Good sources of fiber and other nutrients that play a role in regulating blood pressure and heart health can be hard to find on the grocer's shelf. Read the label! Make sure your whole grains are 100 percent whole.

If the label says "whole grain," look at the ingredient list. If the first ingredient is unbleached wheat flour, that means the product is made mostly of nutrient-depleted white flour. A real, 100 percent whole-grain bread will be heavy in the hand and have a coarser texture than white bread—and it will be labeled "100 percent."

Finding 100 percent whole-grain crackers, cereals, or granola bars is even more difficult. Food companies can be pretty tricky with their labels, making you think a product is good for you when it's not. Again, take the time to read the ingredient list.

Usually the longer the ingredient list, the less likely the product is a real whole food.

There is a chance that even 100 percent whole-wheat products could present a problem for you. Do you suffer with inflammatory bowel syndrome, acid reflux, or joint pain? These may be symptoms of gluten intolerance. The wheat used today was hybridized after World War II to provide higher yields. This high-yield wheat causes health problems for many.

If you think your body may be reacting to this wheat, stop eating it for a couple of weeks to see if you notice a difference in your health. In the meantime, try spelt bread, corn or brown rice pastas, oatmeal for breakfast, and whole grains such as couscous, quinoa, or millet. If you notice that your digestion or joint pain improves after abstaining from wheat, you may want to significantly reduce your wheat intake—or eliminate it from your diet altogether.

Pray together with me.

> *Lord, I eat heart-healthy foods. I am a consistent exerciser. I get my antioxidant nutrients every day. I restrict bad fats and sweets. I am temperate and self-controlled, and keep a calm and undisturbed heart and mind. My heart is healthy. In Jesus's name, amen.*

I am going to make a change today. Here's how:

19 Practice Good Hygiene

*Then turning toward the woman, He said to Simon, Do you
see this woman? When I came into your house, you gave Me
no water for My feet, but she has wet My feet with her tears
and wiped them with her hair.*

—LUKE 7:44

ET'S TALK AGAIN about the most essential drink for getting and staying healthy—fresh, pure, thirst-quenching
water. By now I trust you're drinking more than you ever
have and are enjoying the strength it adds to every tissue and
organ in your body.

Luke 7:44 reveals another powerful property of God's uni-
versal solvent, water. In this verse Jesus says, "You gave Me no
water for My feet, but she has washed My feet with her tears"
(NKJV). Presumably in Jesus's day the roads were dirty and dusty,
and everyone wore sandals. So they needed to wash their feet
much more often than we do today.

In this passage Jesus endorses water as means to cleanse the
body externally. Today many of us have an unlimited supply of
fresh, pure water at our fingertips. We just turn a faucet and
voilà—we have water. What a wonderful blessing to have not
only enough water to drink but also enough to wash our bodies
as often as we like. Thank God for a hot bath and a warm
shower, not to mention the water we need to brush our teeth
and wash our clothes.

Clean water is so readily available in America, you may not
think about the effect cleaning the outside your body has on
your overall health. But it actually makes an enormous impact.

The most common way a cold virus spreads is when we touch something that has been contaminated and then put that contaminated hand to our mouth, nose, or eyes. Contaminating your hands can be as easy as touching a doorknob or a light switch that has been handled recently by an infected person. This transfer of germs and bacteria can be avoided if you simply wash your hands.

Amazingly enough, the first doctor who suggested that physicians wash their hands between patients (a mandatory practice now) was kicked out of his hospital for what was thought to be such a foolish idea.[1] Thousands of years earlier the Old Testament's cleansing laws commanded vigorous hand-washing and the isolation of infected persons, another practice that took thousands of years for the scientific community to embrace. Thank God for water. It cleanses us inside and out.

MAKE A CHANGE TODAY!

Many communities and municipalities today add fluoride to their drinking water. While it has been proven to help prevent cavities (and is useful in mouthwash and toothpaste), fluoride has also been linked to many health problems. Here are just a few:

+ Allergies causing skin rashes, canker sores, gastric distress, headache, joint pain, weakness, visual disturbances, and lethargy[2]

+ Brain issues, including IQ deficits, central nervous system disturbances, and learning and memory problems[3]

+ Bone cancer, namely osteosarcoma, a rare but deadly form of cancer that strikes primarily during the teenage years[4]

- ◆ Kidney damage, as some individuals with kidney disease recovered when switched to fluoride-free water[5]
- ◆ Thyroid dysfunction—according to the US National Research Council, "Several lines of information indicate an effect of fluoride exposure on thyroid function."[6]

The US National Research Council advises that further research be done on the effect of fluoride on various aspects of endocrine function, "particularly with respect to a possible role in the development of several diseases or mental states in the United States."[7] If you're drinking fluoridated water, install a reverse-osmosis filter to remove it from your tap water, or buy water that has been filtered by this process at your local grocery store. Use fluoride to strengthen your teeth and gums but do your best to avoid it in your drinking water.

Let's pray together.

> *I thank You, God, for water—for its availability and its ability to keep me clean. I don't take water for granted. I'm blessed with abundant water for my health. Thank You, Lord Jesus! Amen.*

I am going to make a change today. Here's how:

20 Eat Meat With Care

When they got out on land (the beach), they saw a fire of coals there and fish lying on it [cooking], and bread. Jesus said to them, Bring some of the fish which you have just caught. So Simon Peter went aboard and hauled the net to land, full of large fish, 153 of them; and [though] there were so many of them, the net was not torn. Jesus said to them, Come [and] have breakfast. But none of the disciples ventured or dared to ask Him, Who are You? because they [well] knew that it was the Lord. Jesus came and took the bread and gave it to them, and so also [with] the fish.

—JOHN 21:9–13

SOME HEALTH EXPERTS are convinced that a vegetarian lifestyle is the healthiest. I can certainly agree that for most people decreasing the intake of meat would probably be beneficial. It's also true that God's Word contains several references to the benefits of a vegetable-based diet (Gen. 1:29; Dan. 1:10–16). But does that mean we should all be vegetarians?

The Bible does not teach us to become vegetarians, nor does it tell us to eat 12-ounce steaks at every meal. What should we do? Put simply, we should do what Jesus did. Our food choices will certainly not determine whether we go to heaven. However, if we make all the wrong food choices, we may find ourselves getting to heaven sooner than we thought.

Jesus ate in the Jewish tradition according to the Old Testament dietary laws. The most common meat in Jesus's diet was probably fish.

Today we appreciate the many benefits of the high-quality essential fatty acids found in fish, which are great for the cardiovascular system, brain, and joints. In Leviticus 11:9 the Bible encourages seafood to be eaten only from fish with fins and scales; that is, the clean fish that move through the water.

Forbidden were sea creatures without fins and scales such as the shrimp, crab, and lobster. These are the bottom-dwellers that actually filter the toxins from the water. Pork is forbidden in the same chapter for much the same reason. The pig is a scavenger.

Clean meats included animals that chew the cud, which means they have a literal washing machine of four stomachs that help these animals remove toxins from their system. Although Jesus probably ate clean meats such as cow, deer, and lamb, they were eaten sparingly on feast days and special occasions. Meat is certainly not required at every meal and not even every day, according to the Bible.

MAKE A CHANGE TODAY!

If you are a meat eater, consider selecting grass-fed and free-range meats. Here are four good reasons:

1. Grass-fed and free-range animals don't require the large quantities of antibiotics that are fed to factory-farmed animals. The World Health Organization says the "'overuse and misuse of antibiotics in food animals' is a major source of antibiotic-resistant bacteria that are affecting humans, a major public health crisis."[1]

2. Grass-fed and free-range animals are healthier—and their meat is safer. Cows and chickens weren't meant to eat grains. God designed their stomachs to eat grass. On a diet of grain they produce meat that is more likely to contain parasites and E coli.[2]

3. Meat from grass-fed and free-range animals has less overall fat and less artery-clogging saturated fat. It provides more healthy omega-3 fats, up to four times more vitamin E, and more conjugated linoleic acid, a nutrient that lowers risk of heart disease and cancer.[3]

4. Grass-fed and free-range animals live a happier life. God created animals to be social creatures with an ability to enjoy life. Factory-farmed animals live their lives in pain and without the company of their fellow creatures.[4]

Let's pray together.

Lord, help me to include meat in my diet as Jesus did, sparingly and wisely. In Jesus's name, amen.

I am going to make a change today. Here's how:

21 Conquer Insomnia

When you lie down, you shall not be afraid; yes, you shall lie down, and your sleep shall be sweet.

—PROVERBS 3:24

WE'VE TALKED ABOUT how important it is to let our bodies rest each night in the deep sleep God has promised us. We've also learned how important it is to get the proper amount of sleep by getting to bed on time. But what if you're not getting the results you want when you try to sleep?

We call this habitual sleeplessness insomnia. It can show up as an inability to fall asleep at bedtime or waking up in the night and being unable to return to restful sleep. Whichever the case may be for you, there are alternatives to counting sheep. You need to take a God-pill—Proverbs 3:24 to be specific.

This is God's cure for insomnia. It promises when you lie down you shall not fear; you shall lie down and your sleep shall be sweet. I believe repeating this truth from God's Word can be the foundation of a good night's sleep. Still, as you know, faith without works is dead, so below are some extremely effective tips for ensuring you experience the sweet sleep God promised.

1. One of the best natural ways to ensure a great night's sleep is to make sure you are tired. There is no better way to guarantee this than a consistent exercise program. Do not, however, exercise at bed-time or within a couple of hours before you want

to go to bed. Your body will not have time to relax
properly.[1]

2. Alcohol, tobacco, and caffeine can all interfere with
   restful sleep, as can certain foods. Avoid these at bedtime: bacon, cheese, chocolate, ham, sugar, sausage,
   and tomatoes. These foods all contain a chemical that
   can increase the brain stimulant norepinipherine.[2]
   Certain cold medications and nasal decongestants,
   especially if taken late in the day, also can interfere
   with normal sleep patterns, as can some high blood
   pressure and thyroid medications.[3]

3. Interestingly enough, certain foods containing the
   amino acid tryptophan can help promote sleep. They
   include turkey, figs, dates, yogurt, tuna, whole grains,
   and grapefruit.[4]

4. A healthy sleeping atmosphere can end insomnia for
   some. Other tips: get to bed and wake up at a consistent time each night and morning, take a hot bath
   before bed, turn off the TV when you go to bed, and
   keep the bedroom dark and quiet.[5]

5. Avoid sleeping pills. People who take them regularly
   are 50 percent more like to die in accidents while
   driving or on the job.[6]

A few completely safe and very effective herbs can help nor-
malize your sleeping patterns. Chamomile is a mild sedative
that's safe even for children. My favorite is the much more powerful valerian. Both of these are available in capsule form or as
herbal teas and are best taken at bedtime.[7] It doesn't matter
which of these choices works best for you; they all are tools to
help realize God's promise of a good night's sleep.

MAKE A CHANGE TODAY!

Did you have a problem sleeping last night? Did your schedule keep you from getting a full eight hours of sleep? Do you normally feel fatigued by dinnertime? If you answered yes to any of those questions, then you may want to work a power nap into your day, preferably in the early afternoon. A power nap will help you feel more alert when you wake, but it's not long enough for you to enter the normal sleep cycle, so you won't feel groggy. Want to explore the benefits of power napping? Try these tips:

- **Schedule it**. After lunch is the prime time for a power nap. If you nap after work, don't do it too late in the day. Leave a four- to five-hour window, or you might have trouble getting to sleep at bedtime.
- **Set a timer**. Twenty minutes is optimal. More than thirty minutes could leave you groggy and lethargic the rest of the day.
- **Get comfy**. If possible, find a spot where you can stretch out and elevate your legs. Try to position your head so it tips back at the neck to relieve stress and prevent stiffness.

Here's one more daytime tip that will improve your sleep: break the caffeine habit. Caffeine interferes with a good night's sleep. If you can't totally kick your coffee habit, reserve coffee and other caffeinated beverages for the morning. If you need an afternoon pick-me-up, try a handful of nuts and some fruit. It will give your body an energy boost without disturbing your sleep later on.

Let's pray together.

> *Lord, I am a great sleeper because You give Your beloved rest. I shall lie down, and I shall not fear. I shall lie down and my sleep shall be sweet. In Jesus's name, amen.*

I am going to make a change today. Here's how:

22 Follow a Healthy DIET

*I appeal to you therefore, brethren, and beg of you in view
of [all] the mercies of God, to make a decisive dedication
of your bodies [presenting all your members and faculties]
as a living sacrifice, holy (devoted, consecrated) and well
pleasing to God, which is your reasonable (rational, intelli-
gent) service and spiritual worship.*

—ROMANS 12:1

I WANT TO TALK about diet—but it's not the kind you think.
I am going to take the letters in the word *diet* to help you
remember some important health essentials—tools you'll
need if your goal is to reach and maintain your ideal weight.

+ D is for *decisive*. To be decisive means you know
  exactly what you're doing. Your body is God's, so it
  makes sense to choose to put Him in charge. After
  all, He's the one who wrote your owner's manual,
  the Bible.

+ I is for *inspiration*. Get your inspiration from God's
  Word. It's best to schedule a time each day to read
  the Bible. Ask the Holy Spirit for wisdom and
  direction—just a simple prayer will do—and then
  expect an answer.

+ E is for *eating* and *exercise*. These are the two most
  important factors in determining your weight—and
  your weight is very closely related to overall health.
  Romans 12:1 tells us to present our bodies before
  God, which God counts as spiritual worship. Did

you ever consider that you're worshipping God with the food you put on your plate? And how about going for a brisk walk? God counts that as worship too. Choose God-made foods as much as possible, and aim for thirty minutes of fast-paced walking three to five times a week. Not only will you reach your ideal weight, but you'll also feel much better.

+ *T* is for *thinking*—God's way of thinking, that is. Think of yourself as a brand-new creation. Let old things and habits pass away.

MAKE A CHANGE TODAY!

The food choices in vending machines are rarely nutritious. But if this is where you're heading for lunch, your first inclination might be to choose a muffin or another baked good. However, a look at the product labels reveals that items such as muffins, pies, doughnuts, cinnamon rolls, and even microwave popcorn pack more fat and calories than a candy bar or chips.

How about the "baked" chips? Though one hundred fewer calories than regular chips, they have just as many calories as two Reese's Peanut Butter Cups. Beware of flavored potato and corn chips. They often contain harmful MSG.

The best vending machine selections include peanuts and mixed nuts. While they are high in calories, they give you protein that boosts energy and prevents more cravings. But better still, do your health a favor—plan ahead and bring whole-food snacks from home!

Feeling thirsty? Don't be swayed to quench your thirst with diet soda. Research presented to the American Diabetes Association revealed that drinking diet soda causes unhealthy weight gain. Another study found that aspartame, the artificial sweetener in diet soda, can actually raise blood sugar if you are prone to diabetes.[1]

"Data from this and other prospective studies suggest that the promotion of diet sodas and artificial sweeteners as healthy alternatives may be ill-advised," says Helen P. Hazuda, PhD, chief of clinical epidemiology at the University of Texas Health Science Center San Antonio's School of Medicine. "They may be free of calories but not of consequences."[2]

A third study has shown that people who drink diet sodas every day have more risk for strokes and heart attacks. In addition, soda in general dulls your taste buds, leading you to crave even more sweets.[3] On a recent segment of his television program Dr. Mehmet Oz revealed that diet soda not only causes metabolic syndrome but also damages the bladder and is a leading cause of frequent urination.[4]

The only good beverage choice you'll probably find in the vending machine is water or, if you're lucky, a 100 percent fruit juice or unsweetened green tea. Even if you don't have tons of great options, decide today to make snack choices that will lead to good health.

Let's pray together.

> *I make a decisive choice to dedicate my body to You, Lord. I get my inspiration and instruction from Your Word. I eat God-made foods, which are the best for me. I am a consistent exerciser, and I enjoy it. I think about myself the way You think about me because You promised that being spiritually minded is life and peace to my body. In Jesus's name, amen.*

I am going to make a change today. Here's how:

23 Don't Fear Cancer

Therefore, since these [great] promises are ours, beloved, let us cleanse ourselves from everything that contaminates and defiles body and spirit, and bring [our] consecration to completeness in the [reverential] fear of God.

—2 CORINTHIANS 7:1

TODAY ALMOST EVERYONE has been affected by cancer. Perhaps one of the worst things about cancer is the fear it creates. As we've learned from Proverbs 14:30, fear-based emotions such as anger and jealousy are as "rottenness to the bones" (NKJV). Since the immune system's major cells are formed in the bone marrow, these toxic emotions attack the very efficient and effective mechanism your body has been given to destroy cancer.

Yes, that's right, your immune system is well able to find and destroy cancers in your body by the thousands every day. Cancerous changes occur frequently in the body when an otherwise normal cell starts to divide more rapidly than it should.[1]

Cancer starts out as one simple rebellious cell, which is then recognized by a specialized white blood cell—a T-killer cell—that easily destroys the rogue cell. This is happening in your body right now. That's why I say cancer is really nothing to fear but rather something to educate yourself about. These rebellious cells become a problem when the T-cells are unable to stop their growth.

A cancer diagnosis is certainly not a death sentence. It's an indication that the immune system is not destroying cancer cells as it should. You can do something about that. Interestingly enough the same things you do to help your body fight cancer will also help prevent cancer.

First, detoxify your body. This allows your body to focus on destroying cancer, not on dealing with toxins. A simple way to detoxify is to drink your eight to ten glasses of fresh, purified water every day. Also, make sure you're having at least one bowel movement per day. You can do this by eating a high-fiber diet. Green foods are also great detoxifiers and fight acidity in your body, which promotes cancer.

The other important way to fight cancer is to fortify your immune system. To do this, it is essential that you eat lots of fruits and vegetables and take a high-potency multiple vitamin-mineral supplement. Let's attack cancer and the fear of cancer instead of letting it attack us.

MAKE A CHANGE TODAY!

If you have been diagnosed with cancer, you might consider adopting a macrobiotic diet. One of the most popular alternative lifestyle approaches to cancer, a macrobiotic diet is primarily a vegetarian, whole-foods way of eating, and it includes many of the diet recommendations made to people with cancer.

Scores of remarkable case reports attribute cancer recoveries to a macrobiotic diet. This way of eating also lowers cancer risk. For instance, women who eat macrobiotic diets lower circulating estrogen levels, which can lower risk of breast cancer.[2]

A macrobiotic diet involves eating grains as a staple that is supplemented with local vegetables. Highly processed refined foods and most animal products are avoided. You'd be amazed at how tasty macrobiotic dishes can be!

Macrobiotics also caution against overeating and advises you to chew all food thoroughly before swallowing. For more information on macrobiotics, we recommend *The Hip Chick's Guide to Macrobiotics* and Aveline Kushi's *Complete Guide to Macrobiotic Cooking.*

Let's pray together.

> *Lord, I will keep my body detoxified and strengthen my immune system. I will avoid toxic emotions. My body is a cancer-fighting machine. Cancer cannot live in my body, in Jesus's name, amen.*

I am going to make a change today. Here's how:

24 Laugh Your Way to Wellness

*A happy heart is good medicine and a cheerful mind works
healing, but a broken spirit dries up the bones.*

—PROVERBS 17:22

DID YOU KNOW hearty laughter has positive health benefits? Nehemiah 8:10 says the joy of the Lord is your strength. And, of course, Proverbs 17:22 says "a happy heart is good medicine."

Laughter can help release endorphins into your bloodstream. These natural feel-good neurotransmitters go to work immediately to elevate your mood. Endorphins are also extremely powerful painkillers. Imagine improving your mood and becoming pain-free with something as simple as laughter.

Interestingly enough, the benefits of laughter are not necessarily dependent on how funny something is. Even forced laughter has powerful health benefits. Laughter can help your body destroy cortisol, the major stress hormone that can cause high blood pressure, fat accumulation (especially around the abdomen), and premature aging. That's why I prescribe three belly laughs a day to reverse and prevent sickness and disease. Once again science is discovering what the Bible said so long ago. The breathing patterns associated with laughing can improve oxygenation in the lungs. And a properly oxygenated body produces everything from mental clarity and better brain function to a stronger immune system.

Let's take advantage of this happy highway to health. Laughter is not only free; it also pays enormously healthy dividends and sure beats the alternative. Being overly serious too much of the time is way too stressful on your physical body and sets you up for exhaustion. Little children seem to have this one figured out. The average adult laughs only about ten to fifteen times a day, whereas children laugh more than two hundred times every day.[1] No wonder kids have so much energy and bounce back so quickly from sickness.

So how can we put all this to work for us? Think about what makes you laugh. Is there a certain movie that really makes you giggle? Rent it or, better yet, buy it and start a collection of funny movies. What friend is especially funny? Give him or her a call and schedule some plain, old fun time.

Don't forget those three on-purpose belly laughs every day. Why not have good laugh with each meal? You'll even digest your food better.

Remember, the joy of the Lord is your strength, and a merry heart does good like a medicine. Take this medicine out loud every day and start enjoying these wonderful health benefits. Why don't you have a good laugh right now!

Make a Change Today!

Have a good laugh! Here are a few stories and quotes to help get you started.

A kindergarten teacher was walking around observing her students as they were drawing pictures. When she reached little Vivian, who was working diligently, she asked what she was drawing. Vivian replied, "I'm drawing God." The teacher paused and said, "But no one knows what God looks like." Without looking up from her drawing, the girl replied, "They will in a minute."

The secret of a good sermon is to have a good beginning and a good ending; and to have the two as close together as possible.

—George Burns

Just before she dismissed her class, a Sunday school teacher asked the children to go to church. "And why is it necessary to be quiet in church?" the teacher asked. Jaclyn replied, "Because people are sleeping."

A funeral service is being held in a church for a man who has just passed away. At the end of the service the pallbearers carrying the casket accidentally bump into a wall, jarring the casket. They hear a faint moan. They open the casket and find that the man is actually alive. He lives for ten more years and then dies. A ceremony is again held at the same church, and at the end the pallbearers are again carrying the casket out. As they are walking, the wife calls out, "Watch out for the wall!"

While visiting their grandparents, Donny and Aidon opened the big family Bible. They were fascinated as they fingered through the old pages. Suddenly something fell out. Aidon picked it up and found that it was an old leaf that had been pressed flat between the pages. "Mom, look what I found," he called out. "What have you got there, Aidon?" she asked. With astonishment in his voice, he answered, "I think it's Adam's underwear!"

Let's pray together.

> *Lord, I thank You for the gift of laughter. I have a merry heart, and it does my body good like medicine. I will rejoice in You and gain strength. In Jesus's name, amen.*

I am going to make a change today. Here's how:

25 Drink the Right Water

*Presently, when a woman of Samaria came along to draw
water, Jesus said to her, Give Me a drink.*

—JOHN 4:7

ET'S TALK AGAIN about water. John 4:7 tells of a woman
from Samaria who met Jesus at a well where He was
resting. Jesus said to her, "Give Me a drink." Then in
verse 10 He follows up by telling her, "If you had only known
and had recognized God's gift and Who this is that is saying to
you, Give Me a drink, you would have asked Him [instead] and
He would have given you living water."

In this verse Jesus likens living water to the Spirit of God,
who is the source of life in this world and in the world to come.
Jesus also makes reference in John 4 to our need to continually
drink natural water for the health of our physical bodies. We
should all start our day by saying, as our Creator and Savior did,
"Give me a drink."

When people learn that they need to drink at least eight
glasses of water each day, they ask me what kind of water they
should to drink. Tap water? Well water? What is the best kind
of water? These are great questions. Any kind of water is better
than none at all. Certainly we should avoid contaminated water,
and this is fairly easily and effectively done by drinking water
that has been through a filtration process. Reverse osmosis,
carbon filtration, ozonation, or steam distillation are all accept-
able means for making water healthy for drinking.

Installing some of these filtration systems can be fairly expensive, but I believe it is well worth the cost. If you don't want to

spend money on a built-in filtration system, you should certainly invest the twenty dollars or so needed to purchase one of those do-it-yourself water pitchers with the replaceable carbon gravity filters. You simply pour in water from your faucet and let gravity pull it through the filter. This type of filtration removes more than 98 percent of all contaminants. It is particularly effective at removing the chlorine found in city water.

If I had a choice between municipal water, which contains chlorine, and well water, I would choose well water unless high levels of known contaminants were in the area. Still, in both cases I recommend further filtration.

When it comes to bottled water, certain products are much better than others—and some of the water may not even be filtered. Using your own filtered water is more reliable and less expensive. However, when drinking bottled water, try not to let it sit in the plastic bottle too long and avoid freezing it or letting it heat up. When this happens, dangerous chemicals can leech from the plastic bottle and enter your body as toxins.

Let's thank God for fresh, pure filtered water, which is absolutely essential to keep our bodies clean and detoxified so we can live in divine health.

Make a Change Today!

The only beverage that I recommend in place of water is green tea. Tea is the most consumed beverage in the world, second only to water. And research has found that green tea (made from the *Camellia sinensis plant*) has many health benefits. Made from unfermented tea leaves, green tea contains a high amount of polyphenols, one of many antioxidants that fight damaging compounds in the body that change cells, damage DNA, cause cell death, and promote aging.

In traditional Chinese and Indian medicine, green tea is also used as a stimulant, a diuretic, an astringent, and a means to improve heart health. It is used to treat gas, regulate body temperature and blood sugar, promote digestion, and improve brain function. Studies indicate green tea also may help improve the following health issues:

- Atherosclerosis
- High cholesterol
- Cancer
- Inflammatory bowel disease
- Diabetes
- Liver disease
- Weight loss
- Arthritis
- Symptoms of colds and flu[1]

So in addition to your eight to ten glasses of water, try adding green tea to your diet to promote good health.

Let's pray together.

Lord, I thank You for clean water. I will honor you with my choices by drinking plenty of water every day and healthy beverages such as green tea, in Jesus's name, amen.

I am going to make a change today. Here's how:

26 Get Healthier Inside and Out

So that they should seek God, in the hope that they might feel after Him and find Him, although He is not far from each one of us. For in Him we live and move and have our being; as even some of your [own] poets have said, For we are also His offspring.

—ACTS 17:27–28

ET'S TALK ABOUT how to get healthier inside and out with exercise. Every organ system in your body benefits from regular exercise. Why? Because your body was designed to move!

When not used, muscles will atrophy. That means they shrink away. For instance, after several weeks or months of being immobilized in a cast, a broken leg can shrink to half the size it used to be and have little or no strength.

Having more strength is only one advantage of having bigger muscles. What is the major benefit of having your muscles toned and strong? Believe it or not, having more lean muscle mass in your body makes it much easier to achieve and maintain your ideal weight! I think everyone knows obesity may be the major health problem in the United States. As many as 60 percent to 70 percent of Americans are overweight. Why is this the case? People are taking in more calories in their diets than they are burning off with their muscles.

The two solutions to being overweight are:

1. Decrease caloric intake by cutting back on food
2. Burn more calories

Exercise actually does both. The hormones released when you exercise for stamina and endurance "shrink" the stomach. This means consistent exercisers are less likely to overeat because they tend to get full more quickly. Since you also burn calories when you exercise, you get a double benefit.

With exercise you don't only become healthier on the outside, but you also gain an even greater benefit on the inside. Your immune system is a passive system. It doesn't have a pump. Rather, surrounding muscles squeeze the immune fluids through your body. A sedentary person may move immune fluids through the body only once a day. The exerciser moves these fluids through the body four or five times every day. That means better coverage and protection against every disease. Studies have shown that every hour you exercise can add two hours to your life![1] Now that's an offer you can't refuse!

Make a Change Today!

What one remedy can treat any ailment? Well, exercise helps prevent everything from heart attacks and dementia to diabetes and infection. New research reported by Dr. Beth Levine of the University of Texas Southwestern Medical Center found that exercise promotes autophagy, or "self-eating." This is a mechanism by which surplus, worn-out, or malformed proteins and other cellular components are broken up for scrap and recycled.

Dr. Levine and her team tested their theory by putting mice on a treadmill. They found that the number of autophagosomes in the mice's muscles increased and kept increasing until they had been running for eighty minutes. Long-term, these mice were also less prone to diabetes.[2]

When we recycle parts of ourselves for fuel, we can better prevent diabetes, fight infections, slow the onset of Alzheimer's, and slow aging. Vigorous exercise boosts this recycling process through autophagy. Dr. Levine was so confident about the outcome of her research that she bought herself a treadmill.[3]

Let's pray together.

> *Lord, I am an exerciser. I'm getting healthier on the inside and on the outside because I consistently exercise. I'm adding years to my life with exercise, in Jesus's name, amen.*

I am going to make a change today. Here's how:

27 Improve Your Memory

*For God did not give us a spirit of timidity...but [He has
given us a spirit] of power and of love and of calm and
well-balanced mind and discipline and self-control.*

—2 TIMOTHY 1:7

IS IT TRUE that as you age your memory automatically gets
weaker? If you live long enough, will you inevitably experience presenile dementia, senility, and even Alzheimer's disease? You may be as surprised as I was to learn that leading
experts in neuroscience have discovered that you do not have
to expect memory loss and brain malfunction no matter what
your age.

Doctors used to believe you were born with all the brain
cells you'll ever have, that you lose about ten thousand of them
a day, and that by the time you're around sixty-five years old you
should expect mental deficits. Not true! We actually have the
ability to repair existing brain cells, build new neuronal path-
ways, and create new brain cells even in our mature years. The
exciting part is you can take action to help your brain function
efficiently and *improve* as you age.

This little mnemonic for the word *brain* outlines what you
can do to increase mental functioning and avoid Alzheimer's
and dementia altogether!

- *B* is for *B vitamins*. These vitamins fight stress, especially in brain cells. I recommend a multivitamin
  supplement with all the B vitamins included.

- *R* reminds us to *restrict calories.* People who eat less tend to have better brain function. Of course, you need adequate calories, but fasting one day a week can really improve mental acuity. Skipping dessert and second helpings certainly won't hurt.

- *A* stands for *antioxidants.* The ACES—vitamins A, C and E, and the trace mineral selenium—help the brain fight free-radical damage, which if left unchecked increases the aging rate of brain cells. Make sure your multivitamin-mineral supplement contains adequate antioxidants.

- *I* is a reminder to *increase oxygenation.* A properly oxygenated brain is a healthy brain. Exercise is key here, as is staying mentally active by exercising your brain with new challenges daily. Even reading a daily Bible verse can help in this area.

- *N* is for *nutrients* (brain food). Make sure you are getting the essential fatty acids found in nuts, seeds, and fish. The best eating plan for a strong brain is getting plenty of God-made foods.

MAKE A CHANGE TODAY!

Below are eight ways to boost your brainpower.

1. **Try a taste test.** When you eat, try to figure out the individual ingredients in your meal.
2. **Take a cooking class.** Cooking uses all five of your senses, and each uses a different part of your brain.
3. **Memorize lists.** Make a list—for groceries, to-dos, Christmas gifts, etc.—and memorize it. An hour later see how many items you can remember.

4. **Draw a map**. When you get home from visiting a new destination, draw a map of the area.

5. **Work on hand-eye coordination**. Try knitting, drawing, painting, or assembling a puzzle.

6. **Do the math**. Figure out math problems without pencil, paper, computer, or calculator.

7. **Visualize words in your head**.

8. **Take music lessons**. Learning to play a musical instrument boosts brain skills.[1]

Let's pray together.

Lord, my brain is strong. I have a great memory, and it's getting better every day. I exercise my brain and my body, and I get the nutrients I need for a sound mind. In Jesus's name, amen.

I am going to make a change today. Here's how:

28 Practice Fasting

And whenever you are fasting, do not look gloomy and sour and dreary like the hypocrites, for they put on a dismal countenance, that their fasting may be apparent to and seen by men. Truly I say to you, they have their reward in full already.

—Matthew 6:16

BELIEVE FASTING IS one of the most underutilized health-promoting modalities in existence. God's Word even makes it very clear that fasting is expected! In Matthew 6 Jesus says, "When you pray" (v. 5), and we all know we need to pray. He also says, "When you give" (v. 3), and we know the importance of giving. Then in the same chapter Jesus said, "When you fast" (v. 17). So the issue is not whether you *should* fast but *how* and *when* you should fast.

Fasting simply means to go without food for a period of time. But fasting is not just a hunger strike! When the Bible speaks of fasting, it always talks about fasting *and* prayer. When you use the time you'd normally spend eating and preparing meals in the Word and prayer, you make your fasting experience even more valuable.

Isaiah 58 promises that fasting will produce a number of results. First, our health will spring forth speedily (v. 8). Imagine a quicker recovery from sickness or disease because you take advantage of prayer and fasting. Second, fasting will make your bones strong (v. 11). And you know the bone marrow is where many of the cells of the immune system are formed. Third, fasting will help you hear the voice of the Lord better. Isaiah 58:11 promises that the Lord will guide you continually.

I believe you should make it your goal to fast at least one day per week. If you've never fasted before, start by fasting just one meal, then two, and finally twenty-four hours. A water-only fast is a most powerful fast, but if you need to drink a little fruit or vegetable juice to get you through, that's OK. At the change of seasons you may even want to try a two- or three-day fast to experience even more spiritual and physical benefits.

Make a Change Today!

Cardiac researchers from the Intermountain Medical Center Heart Institute found that routine, periodic fasting is good for your health and your heart. They discovered that fasting lowers risk of coronary artery disease and diabetes while also lowering blood cholesterol levels. Diabetes and high cholesterol can lead to coronary heart disease, which is the leading cause of death among men and women in America. Fasting also helps maintain healthy triglyceride, weight, and blood sugar levels, which are other factors in heart health.[1]

"Fasting causes hunger or stress. In response, the body releases more cholesterol, allowing it to utilize fat as a source of fuel instead of glucose. This decreases the number of fat cells in the body," says Benjamin D. Horne, PhD, MPH, of the Intermountain Medical Center Heart Institute. "This is important because the fewer fat cells a body has, the less likely it will experience insulin resistance, or diabetes."[2]

This recent study also confirmed earlier findings about the effects of fasting on human growth hormone (HGH), a metabolic protein. "HGH works to protect lean muscle and metabolic balance, a response triggered and accelerated by fasting."[3]

The benefits of fasting far outweigh the short-term discomfort.

This spiritual discipline will produce positive and lasting health results.

Let's pray together.

> *Thank You, Lord, for Your promises of better health and a closer walk with You through prayer and fasting. Help me to get started on this wonderful habit this week! In Jesus's name, amen.*

I am going to make a change today. Here's how:

29 Meet God's Answer to Depression

To grant [consolation and joy] to those who mourn in Zion—
to give them an ornament (a garland or diadem) of beauty
instead of ashes, the oil of joy instead of mourning, the gar-
ment [expressive] of praise instead of a heavy, burdened,
and failing spirit—that they may be called oaks of righteous-
ness [lofty, strong, and magnificent, distinguished for upright-
ness, justice, and right standing with God], the planting of the
Lord, that He may be glorified.

—ISAIAH 61:3

DEPRESSION IS A whole-body illness. It can affect the way you eat, sleep, and react to things around you. Changes in appetite or energy level, loss of interest in hobbies, and feelings of worthlessness and inadequacy are not uncommon. The causes of depression are many and varied. It may be triggered by stress, poor diet, lack of exercise, a traumatic life event, or any serious physical disorder.

The most common type of depression is a chronic low-grade depression called dysthymia. This type of depression is not usually disabling but simply keeps a person from normal social interaction and enjoying life. Research has shown this type of depression is often associated with negative thinking patterns.

Some forms of depression require a doctor's care. But God has an answer to depression. And in some cases you can beat depression when you M-E-E-T it on His terms.

+ **Make your request known to God.** Philippians 4:6 says not to worry about anything but, instead, to tell God what you desire. You must want to be free from depression enough to make the necessary changes. Start by asking God to free you from oppression (Ps. 62:10) and give you His joy (Prov. 15:23), which is your strength (Ps. 28:7). Use your mouth to request this out loud. Remember, the tongue has the power of life and death (Prov. 18:21).

+ **Exercise.** This increases endorphins, those feel-good neurotransmitters in your brain. Exercise also increases circulation to your brain, which helps to balance your mood and increase your alertness.

+ **Eat foods that fight depression.** God-made foods are especially beneficial here: fruits, vegetables, and whole grains—raw whenever possible. Nuts and seeds contain essential fatty acids critical for brain function. The best source of protein is fish. It is very important that you avoid junk foods and processed foods with artificial colors, flavors, or preservatives, as these foods lack the nutrients that will help strengthen your body.

+ **Think praise and thank God.** Isaiah 61:3 says God has given you the garment of praise for the spirit of heaviness, which is another way of describing depression. You put on the garment of praise by putting into practice Psalm 103:2, which reminds us to "bless the LORD, O my soul [the mind, will, and emotions], and forget not all His benefits" (NKJV).

MAKE A CHANGE TODAY!

While exercise might be the last thing you feel like doing when you're depressed, it should be the first thing in your treatment plan. According to the Mayo Clinic, "Research on anxiety, depression and exercise shows that the psychological and physical benefits of exercise can also help reduce anxiety and improve mood.... Working out can definitely help you relax and make you feel better. Exercise may also help keep anxiety and depression from coming back once you're feeling better."[1]

Exercise relieves depression and anxiety two ways: physically and mentally.

Physically

- Exercise releases feel-good brain chemicals, neurotransmitters, and endorphins.
- Exercise reduces immune system chemicals that deepen depression.
- Exercise increases body temperature, which has a calming effect.[2]

Mentally

- You gain confidence because you feel successful and improve your appearance.
- You take your focus off your problems.
- You increase social interaction when you go to the gym or walk around the block.[3]

By attacking it spiritually and physically, you can beat depression and experience God's lasting joy and peace.

Let's pray together.

> *Lord, I'm meeting Your answer for depression by making my request for Your joy. I eat properly and exercise to improve my mood. I put on the garment of praise, which destroys the spirit of heaviness and depression. In Jesus's name, amen.*

I am going to make a change today. Here's how:

30 Unlock Wellness With the Ten Keys That Cure

Be not wise in your own eyes; reverently fear and worship the Lord and turn [entirely] away from evil. It shall be health to your nerves and sinews, and marrow and moistening to your bones.

—PROVERBS 3:7–8

Now I WANT to summarize and simplify much of what we've been talking about throughout this book. What is the basic Bible blueprint for our health? The answer is found in our key scripture, Proverbs 3:7–8. You've read many times that the bones are where the cells of the immune system are formed. So what must you do to receive "health to your nerves and sinews, and marrow...to your bones"? Fear the Lord and depart from evil. In simple English that means knowing and doing what's right according to Scripture.

In searching the Bible, I've found support for ten simple keys that will have a tremendous positive effect on your health. Let's go over those ten keys as a review and a reminder of what God says is good for your health.

1. **Learn to relax.** You know stress can be the number one enemy of your immune system. This means you must cast all your cares on God (1 Pet. 5:7) and ask Him to give you the divine health He promises.

2. **Get to bed on time**. Sleep is restoration time. It's impossible to stay healthy without adequate rest.

3. **Exercise regularly.** Exercise provides so many health benefits—everything from mood

improvement to immune fluid movement to increasing metabolism for ideal weight. Remember—move it and improve it!

4. **Breathe fresh air**. Oxygen is the most essential nutrient for every cell, and you need it every second of your life. Infections and cancer hate oxygen.

5. **Go outside when the sun is out**. A moderate amount of sunshine converts the cholesterol in your skin to vitamin D, which helps strengthen bones.

6. **Eat your fruits**. They are God's sweet, healthy treats.

7. **Eat your vegetables**. Veggies are the very foundation of good health, especially raw ones.

8. **Eat whole grains**. Anything less than 100 percent whole grain is not worth putting inside God's temple.

9. **Eat meat sparingly and choose white over dark**. Fish, chicken, and turkey are the best options, with fish being the healthiest choice.

10. **Drink water**. It's what you are made of. After reading the tips in this book, I know you won't forget the detoxifying, cleansing, hydrating, and other health-promoting benefits of fresh purified water.

I encourage you to apply these ten principles today. God wants you to have good health. I am standing in agreement with you that you will experience the perfect well-being God has designed for you and fulfill the number of days He has planned for your life as you follow His simple pathway for health.

Let's pray together.

> *Lord, I'm going to learn to relax the way You want me to and get to bed on time. I'm going to start and continue to exercise. I will breathe fresh air when the sun's out. My diet is based on God-made fruit, vegetables, and whole grains. I choose white meats and drink what I'm mostly made of—water. I will drink eight to ten glasses of fresh, pure water every day. I expect to enjoy divine health all the days of my life, and the number of my days will be fulfilled. In Jesus's name, amen.*

I am going to make a change today. Here's how:

Notes

2—LEARN TO RELAX

1. Daniel Goleman, "Relaxation: Surprising Benefits Detected," *New York Times*, May 13, 1986, http://www.nytimes.com/1986/05/13/science/relaxation-surprising-benefits-detected.html?pagewanted=all (accessed November 13, 2012).

3—DRINK MORE WATER

1. Stan Moore, *Living Well by Water* (Hattiesburg, MS: M&M Publishing, 2001).
2. Angela Ogunjimi, "The Average Consumption of Water Per Day," LiveStrong.com, August 11, 2012, http://www.livestrong.com/article/338496-the-average-consumption-of-water-per-day/ (accessed November 11, 2012).
3. US Geological Survey, "The Water in You," http://ga.water.usgs.gov/edu/propertyyou.html (accessed November 11, 2012).
4. Science Dailey, "Drink Water to Curb Weight Gain? Clinical Trial Confirms Effectiveness of Simple Appetite Control Method," http://www.sciencedaily.com/releases/2010/08/100823142929.htm (accessed November 11, 2012).
5. WebMD, "Sodas and Your Health: Risks Debated," http://www.webmd.com/diet/features/sodas-and-your-health-risks-debated (accessed November 11, 2012).

4—TRY THE GENESIS DIET

1. *Targum Onkelos*, Genesis 2:7, http://targum.info/pj/pjgen1-6.htm (accessed December 17, 2012).
2. The World's Healthiest Foods, "Flaxseeds," http://whfoods.org/genpage.php?tname=foodspice&dbid=81 (accessed November 11, 2012).
3. The World's Healthiest Foods, "Sesame Seeds," http://whfoods.org/genpage.php?tname=foodspice&dbid=84 (accessed November 11, 2012).
4. The World's Healthiest Foods, "Pumpkin Seeds," http://whfoods.org/genpage.php?tname=foodspice&dbid=82 (accessed November 11, 2012); Exercise4WeightLostt.com, "Benefits of Pumpkin and Pumpkin Seeds," http://www.exercise4weightloss.com/benefits-of-pumpkin.html (accessed November 11, 2012).
5. The World's Healthiest Foods, "Sunflower Seeds," http://whfoods.org/genpage.php?tname=foodspice&dbid=57 (accessed November 11, 2012).

6. The World's Healthiest Foods, "Cumin Seeds," http://whfoods.org/genpage.php?tname=foodspice&dbid=91 (accessed November 11, 2012).

5—GET TO BED ON TIME

1. National Sleep Foundation, "How Much Sleep Do We Really Need?" http://www.sleepfoundation.org/article/how-sleep-works/how-much-sleep-do-we-really-need (accessed November 11, 2012).
2. Ibid.
3. Ibid.

6—BEGIN TO EXERCISE

1. Len Kravitz, "Exercise Motivation: What Starts and Keeps People Exercising?", http://www.unm.edu/~lkravitz/Article%20folder/ExerciseMot.pdf (accessed November 13, 2012).
2. Ibid.

7—CALM YOUR MIND

1. Babes Tan-Magkalas, "Praying Hands Calms the Mind," TheHolyStory.com, http://theholystory.com/praying-hands-calms-the-mind.html (accessed November 11, 2012).

8—CLEAN THE INSIDE OF YOUR BODY

1. Mayo Clinic, "Dehydration: Risk Factors," January 7, 2011, http://www.mayoclinic.com/health/dehydration/DS00561/DSECTION=risk-factors (accessed November 11, 2012).

10—SLEEP BETTER AND LIVE MORE PRODUCTIVELY

1. Phyllis A. Balch, *Prescription for Nutritional Healing*, fourth edition (New York: Penguin Group USA, 2006), 528. Viewed online at Google Books.
2. The Institute for Natural Healing, "Why Sleeping Pills Only Buy You 11 Minutes of Sleep Each Night," October 19, 2011, http://naturalhealthdossier.com/2011/10/why-sleeping-pills-only-buy-you-11-minutes-of-sleep-each-night/ (accessed November 11, 2012).
3. Ibid.
4. National Sleep Foundation, "Can't Sleep? What to Know About Insomnia," http://www.sleepfoundation.org/article/sleep-related-problems/insomnia-and-sleep (accessed December 17, 2012).

11—WATCH YOUR WORDS

1. R. Douglas Fields, "Sticks and Stones—Hurtful Words Damage the Brain," *Psychology Today*, October 30, 2010, http://www.psychologytoday.com/blog/the-new-brain/201010/sticks-and-stones-hurtful-words-damage-the-brain (accessed November 11, 2012).

12—LET GO OF ENVY, JEALOUSY, AND ANGER

1. PR Newswire, "Jealousy Paralyzes Creativity, Productivity, and Relationships, Says Stress Relief Expert Lauren E. Miller," July 12, 2011, http://www.prnewswire.com/news-releases/jealousy-paralyzes-creativity-productivity-and-relationships-says-stress-relief-expert-lauren-e-miller-125405253.html (accessed November 11, 2012).
2. Ibid.

14—LIVE LEAN

1. IDEA Health and Fitness Association, "Why Women Need Weight Training," http://www.ideafit.com/fitness-library/weight-training-for-women (accessed November 11, 2012).
2. Bastyr Center for Natural Health, "Smaller Entrées Help Kids Eat More Fruits and Veggies," http://www.bastyrcenter.org/content/view/2366/ (accessed November 11, 2012)

16—THINK WELL AND BE WELL

1. Erica Goode, "Power of Positive Thinking May Have a Health Benefit, Study Says," *New York Times*, September 2, 2003, http://www.nytimes.com/2003/09/02/health/power-of-positive-thinking-may-have-a-health-benefit-study-says.html (accessed November 12, 2012).
2. Ibid.

19—PRACTICE GOOD HYGIENE

1. Encyclopedia Britannica, "Ignaz Philipp Semmelweis" http://www.britannica.com/EBchecked/topic/534198/Ignaz-Philipp-Semmelweis (accessed November 12, 2012).
2. Fluoride Action Network, "Hypersensitivity," http://www.fluoridealert.org/issues/health/hypersensitivity/ (accessed November 12, 2012).
3. Fluoride Action Network, "Brain," http://www.fluoridealert.org/issues/health/brain/ (accessed November 12, 2012).
4. Fluoride Action Network, "Cancer," http://www.fluoridealert.org/issues/health/cancer/ (accessed November 12, 2012).
5. Fluoride Action Network, "Kidney Disease," http://www.fluoridealert.org/issues/health/kidney/ (accessed November 12, 2012).
6. Fluoride Action Network, "Thyroid," http://www.fluoridealert.org/issues/health/thyroid/ (accessed November 12, 2012).
7. Ibid.

20—EAT MEAT WITH CARE

1. Natural Resources Defense Council, "Top 10 Reasons to Eat Grass-Fed Meat," http://www.nrdc.org/living/eatingwell/top-10-reasons-eat-grass-fed-meat.asp (accessed November 12, 2012).

2. Ibid.
3. Ibid.
4. Ibid.

21—CONQUER INSOMNIA

1. Balch, *Prescription for Nutritional Healing*, fourth edition, 527. Viewed online at Google Books.
2. Ibid.
3. National Sleep Foundation, "Sleep Aids and Insomnia," http://www .sleepfoundation.org/article/sleep-related-problems/sleep-aids-and-insomnia (accessed November 12, 2012).
4. Balch, *Prescription for Nutritional Healing*, fourth edition, 527. Viewed online at Google Books.
5. Ibid., 527
6. Ibid., 529.
7. Ibid., 527.

22—FOLLOW A HEALTHY DIET

1. ScienceDaily, "Waistlines in People, Glucose Levels in Mice Hint at Sweeteners' Effects: Related Studies Point to the Illusion of the Artificial," June 28, 2011, http://www.sciencedaily.com/releases/2011/06/110627183944 .htm (accessed November 12, 2012).
2. Ibid.
3. Steven Morris, "Sugary Drinks Dull Taste Buds, Study Claims," *The Guardian*, June 9, 2011, http://www.guardian.co.uk/lifeandstyle/2011/ jun/09/sugary-drinks-dull-tastebuds-study?CMP=twt_fd (accessed November 12, 2012).
4. Pat Howard, "Dr Oz: Artificial Sweeteners & Sugar Substitutes Cause Bladder Damage?", DrOzFans.com, October 8, 2012, http://www .drozfans.com/dr-oz-diet/dr-oz-artificial-sweeteners-sugar-substitutes-cause -bladder-damage/ (accessed November 12, 2012).

23—DON'T FEAR CANCER

1. American Cancer Society, "Questions People Ask About Cancer," http:// www.cancer.org/cancer/cancerbasics/questions-people-ask-about-cancer (accessed November 12, 2012).
2. Lawrence H. Kushi, Joan E. Cunningham, James R. Hebert, Robert H. Lerman, Elisa V. Bandera, and Jane Teas, "The Macrobiotic Diet in Cancer," *Journal of Nutrition* 131, no. 11 (November 1, 2001): http:// jn.nutrition.org/content/131/11/3056S.full (accessed November 12, 2012).

24—LAUGH YOUR WAY TO WELLNESS

1. US Department of Health and Human Services, Substance Abuse & Mental Health Services Administration, "Humor and Kids," http://bblocks.samhsa.gov/family/talkingListening/Dhumandkids.aspx (accessed November 12, 2012).

25—DRINK THE RIGHT WATER

1. University of Maryland Medical Center, "Green Tea," http://www.umm.edu/altmed/articles/green-tea-000255.htm (accessed November 12, 2012).

26—GET HEALTHIER INSIDE AND OUT

1. American Heart Association, "Physical Activity Improves Quality of Life," http://www.heart.org/HEARTORG/GettingHealthy/PhysicalActivity/StartWalking/Physical-activity-improves-quality-of-life_UCM_307977_Article.jsp (accessed November 12, 2012).
2. UT Southwestern Medical Center Newsroom, "Health Benefits of Exercise May Depend on Cellular Degradation, Researchers Report," January 20, 2012, http://www.utsouthwestern.edu/newsroom/news-releases/year-2012/levine-autophagy-nature.html (accessed November 12, 2012).
3. *The Economist*, "Worth all the Sweat," January 21, 2012, http://www.economist.com/node/21543129 (accessed November 12, 2012).

27—IMPROVE YOUR MEMORY

1. Linda Malone, "Brain Exercises That Boost Memory," *Everyday Health*, September 18, 2008, http://www.everydayhealth.com/longevity/mental-fitness/brain-exercises-for-memory.aspx (accessed November 12, 2012).

28—PRACTICE FASTING

1. Intermountain Medical Center, "Study Finds Routine Periodic Fasting Is Good for Your Health and Your Heart" April 3, 2011, http://www.eurekalert.org/pub_releases/2011-04/imc-sfr033111.php (accessed November 13, 2012).
2. Ibid.
3. Ibid.

29—MEET GOD'S ANSWER TO DEPRESSION

1. Mayo Clinic Staff, "Depression and Anxiety: Exercise Eases Symptoms," MayoClinic.com, October 1 2011, http://www.mayoclinic.com/health/depression-and-exercise/MH00043 (accessed November 13, 2012).
2. Ibid.
3. Ibid.

About the Author

DON VERHULST, MD, received his BS in zoology at the University of Michigan in 1978 and his MD from Wayne State University School of Medicine in 1982. As he began to study the Bible from a physician's perspective, the Lord showed him the divine health principles found in His Word. Dr. Don decided that the Bible was the best physiology textbook he ever studied—accurate in every detail and filled with promise after promise about health and healing. He realized that God has a marvelous health plan for each of His children— He gives us many amazing keys to good health right in the pages of His Word!

In response to God's call, Dr. Don lectures in schools, churches, and businesses. He and his wife, Susan Krews VerHulst, host their own weekly TV program, *Hope for Your Health*, which is broadcast throughout North America on the TCT Network. Dr. Don and Susan also appear as regular guests on *The Jim Bakker Show* and radio programs broadcast across the nation. Because of his passion for writing and performing music, Dr. Don often shares his songs on health and healing when he teaches.

Dr. Don's first full-length book, *Ten Keys That Cure: Bible Truths for Better Health Today*, enjoyed great success. A revised and updated edition, *Do This and Live Healthy: 10 Simple Keys That Cure* was published by Siloam in 2012. Dr. Don's children's book, *Count to Ten and Be Healthy With Dr. Don*, has quickly become a favorite in Christian homes across the nation.

When Dr. Don and Susan are not busy traveling or lecturing, they enjoy spending time with their four children, Donnie, Aidon, Jaclyn, and Vivian.

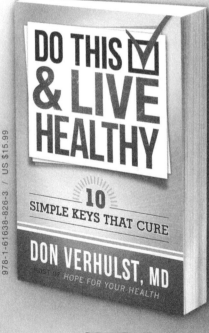